Contested Illness in Context

What makes a disease real? Why is it that patients with chronic fatigue syndrome or fibromyalgia are doubted when they say they are in pain, and cannot access the same benefits of patient-hood that others can? What defines the limits of our belief and, ultimately, compassion, when it comes to disease?

These are the questions approached in this book, which draws upon patients' experiences and situates them among a diverse set of literatures, from the history and philosophy of medicine to the sociology of health and disease. The question of a patient's identity and their understanding of disease is often assumed to emerge from their relationship with healthcare, but the case is made here that other, inter-personal factors are more salient. What a patient with a contested illness comes up against is not simply a medical categorisation – it is a prevailing notion of disease across society, and one they struggle to assimilate themselves into.

Contested Illness in Context will appeal to students and researchers interested in fields such as the history and philosophy of medicine, the sociology of health and illness, medical anthropology, or disease and illness generally. It may also interest patients and doctors who struggle with difficult medical cases.

Harry Quinn Schone brings clarity to the blurry edges of disease, where biology and social factors collide. He is particularly interested in the epistemic conflicts present in contested illnesses, and the consequences of such tussles on patients.

Routledge Studies in the Sociology of Health and Illness

Recovery, Mental Health and Inequality
Chinese Ethnic Minorities as Mental Health Service Users
Lynn Tang

Fertility, Health and Lone Parenting
European Contexts
Edited by Fabienne Portier-Le Cocq

Transnationalising Reproduction
Third Party Conception in a Globalised World
Edited by Róisín Ryan Flood and Jenny Gunnarsson Payne

Public Health, Personal Health and Pills
Drug Entanglements and Pharmaceuticalised Governance
Kevin Dew

Dementia as Social Experience
Valuing Life and Care
Edited by Gaynor Macdonald and Jane Mears

Injecting Bodies in More-than-Human Worlds
Mediating Drug-Body-World Relations
Fay Dennis

Contested Illness in Context
An Interdisciplinary Study in Disease Definition
Harry Quinn Schone

For more information about this series, please visit: https://www.routledge.com/Routledge-Studies-in-the-Sociology-of-Health-and-Illness/book-series/RSSHI

Contested Illness in Context

An Interdisciplinary Study in Disease Definition

Harry Quinn Schone

Routledge
Taylor & Francis Group
LONDON AND NEW YORK

First published 2019
by Routledge
2 Park Square, Milton Park, Abingdon, Oxon OX14 4RN

and by Routledge
605 Third Avenue, New York, NY 10017

First issued in paperback 2020

Routledge is an imprint of the Taylor & Francis Group, an informa business

British Library Cataloguing-in-Publication Data
A catalogue record for this book is available from the British Library

Library of Congress Cataloging-in-Publication Data
A catalog record has been requested for this book

ISBN 13: 978-0-367-73001-7 (pbk)
ISBN 13: 978-0-367-02644-8 (hbk)

Typeset in Times New Roman
by Taylor & Francis Books

MIX
Paper from responsible sources
FSC™ C013985
www.fsc.org

Printed in the United Kingdom
by Henry Ling Limited

For George

Contents

Acknowledgements

Thanks, first and foremost, to the patients who so kindly gave their time to talk to me, and without whom there would be no book. Thanks, too, to Brendan Clarke, to whom I presumably now owe some more whisky. Finally, thanks to my wife, Ieva, for everything she has done, past and present, and for the truly wondrous person that she is.

Pain, as a symptom of the problematic, frequently is.

Drew Leder

Introduction

This work will look in detail at the philosophical context that frames the ways contested illnesses are experienced and understood by patients in the early 21st century. The key focus of this book is to trace with greater accuracy – and, more importantly, greater reference to lived experience – the contours of belief and assumption which provide us with our collective map of disease.

There is not an easy category in which to place this work. It is partly historical, in that I utilise the writings of historians to provide insight into our contemporary concerns and it is impossible to understand the current state of disease beliefs prevalent across society without paying attention to the historical processes which have deposited a way of viewing and feeling disease into our collective subconscious. It is also, in part, sociological, in that I borrow from sociology ways of listening to and observing illness. Furthermore, sociology has provided us with the most substantial critique of the biomedical view of the body by highlighting the cases in which it is inappropriate and ill-fitted, and to this research I shall refer extensively. And though this work is clearly interdisciplinary, it is most of all philosophical. Throughout my discussions I return time and time again to fundamental questions of conceptualisation: what do we expect a disease to look like? What prevailing notions dictate the way we are allowed to, expect ourselves to be, and in some way *are* ill? To whom does epistemic authority over these ideas belong to and originate from?

I mean these questions to be read in a philosophical sense as attempts to probe beneath the surface of our *reaction* to disease. In other words, how does a sick person understand their illness metaphysically, how do people around them approach it and what are the consequences of these beliefs?

My argument, to be expounded greatly in the following pages, can be summarised as follows. Many, if not all, of the different concepts that philosophers associate with illness suffer a loss of clarity under stringent investigation, and it is doubtful whether they are theoretically resilient enough to be relied upon when constructing a coherent theory of disease. What does emerge from their examination, however, is a more general impression, a broad framework through which it is possible to view the way disease is mediated and understood. From this we are able to envisage what shape illness takes on unconsciously, implicitly, in the imagination, the ways in which it is expected to show itself and the ways in which people and institutions are expected to relate to it. In short, the way disease *operates* in our society.

With this idea in mind, we consider 'contested illnesses', those which do not conform to our vision, those which lie outside of our expectations. The aim is not to show that people with these conditions are 'really' ill, or are deserving of sympathy, though this is in my view certainly true. Rather, I want to put it that we intuitively categorise disease according to certain predispositions, and when we encounter a phenomenon which contradicts these prejudices, a gap opens up between our expectations of disease and the condition itself, the thing before us. This gap creates a tension, a painful distance, but it is not purely theoretical. On the contrary, it is precisely in this space that harm occurs. This is found institutionally, in the form of welfare disputes or dismissals from employment; interpersonally in the breakdown of trust and respect in a marriage; psychologically in the self-doubt and depression of an ill person who lacks an approved way of deciphering the way they feel in their body.

My thought is that while much attention has been given to both analysing concepts related to disease and to investigating the relationship between institutions and individuals of authority and patients, little focus has been granted philosophically to the ways in which we all – as friends, family members, colleagues, patients – contribute to and constitute the experience and meaning of disease. In other words, I think that the quest to define disease, to map the landscape of the doctor/patient relationship, to understand how patients interact with their condition as described to them institutionally has eschewed broader questions about the underlying metaphysical assumptions that exist in the minds of clinicians and non-specialists alike. Essentially, I say that we cannot define disease, but we can look at the ways it *is* defined, who is doing the defining, on what basis they make that distinction, and what the effects of such a demarcation are.[1]

Caveats, of course, abound. This book does not aim to answer any questions of medical science. What this work tries to achieve instead is an illumination of the way in which the medical aspects of a disease: diagnosis, labelling, treatment and so on intersect with social beliefs about sickness and contribute to the manifestation of illness in an individual, both in terms of their symptoms and how they understand them, but also in terms of how those symptoms are greeted by others. Medicine is therefore just one of many components which have an effect on our idea of a disease, on our acceptance

1 These sound like very sociological questions. But what I am trying to get close to is outlining the unconscious, seemingly intuitive set of beliefs and expectations that cause a person to look at another and say 'you are sick' or 'you are not ill', a process that I think too obscure and too internal to be classified as an object of sociological inquiry.

or rejection of a certain set of phenomena as a disease concept. It is afforded no special status in this analysis.

However, it should be highlighted that contested illnesses would benefit from more clarity in this (medical) and other areas, and I hope that my work on this topic might inspire others in different fields to approach these difficult questions. Doctors, psychiatrists, health researchers, sociologists and other philosophers will find some interesting topics discussed here and may wish to pursue them further within their own specialities.

Also to be noted is that the overriding emphasis of this work is not to generate universals or to speak in grand terms, but rather to examine the specific and draw from it certain insights which may tentatively be said to represent *something* if not nearly *everything* that can be said about the topic. As such, it is difficult to see how the conclusions of the work presented below could be extended confidently beyond a Western context, and even then, a heavy bias towards UK and US sources is prevalent.

Furthermore, consistent with my stated commitment to specificity, this book is anchored in a precise time and place, and makes no claims to represent anything more than a snapshot of a particular moment. I take a lead from Floridi (2011, p. 12), who writes that any 'timeless' philosophy is a stagnant one. This is a book about contested disease as it is lived and understood here and now, and nowhere else.

Part I

A language of disease

Chapter 1

Contested illnesses

Introduction

By choosing to look at contested illnesses I have quite deliberately picked a group of diseases that live within the crux of many philosophical problems.[1] These are the conditions unaccounted for by biomedical models, the ailments that debilitate and destroy without explanation or acceptance. They straddle both the physical and the mental, but share a sense of dislocation; doctors are not trained to help their non-specific pain, partners are not naturally inclined to sympathise and institutions are not willing to accept them as genuine. They are precisely those illnesses which disconnect from our expectations of disease, and in the gap created lay bare our previous assumptions about what a disease is or what is necessary for someone to be sick. But is this a useful category, or indeed a category at all? Is it possible to adequately define a contested illness?

In this chapter I will discuss the features of a contested illness, starting from Swoboda's (2005) definition and using the contrasting examples of asthma and chronic fatigue syndrome to sketch a more complete outline of the concept. I will also discuss how one very common, almost essential aspect of contested illnesses – their chronic nature – lends itself to philosophical evaluation.

Contested illnesses

At first glance (and this is the point), it might seem that there are so many ways that a disease could be considered 'contested' that describing one as such becomes virtually meaningless. However, in this section I aim to show that it is possible to demarcate contested illness in a meaningful way. Though it's true that many diseases contain disputed elements, the conditions I write about in this work are figures of doubt in their entirety – the type of contestation that occurs is fundamental not specific. They are illnesses that

1 Some examples of contested illness include fibromyalgia, chronic fatigue syndrome, chronic Lyme disease, toxic mould syndrome, Gulf War syndrome, sick building syndrome, multiple chemical sensitivity and silicone breast implant disease.

appear to us not as controversial because we don't know their exact mechanism or which drugs are most effective at treating them but because in some sense we suspect them to *not exist*. They are, in my terminology, *ontologically* contested. But first, in what ways might a disease be considered contested and why are these criteria often inadequate in the making of a bona fide contested disease?

Illnesses can be disputed clinically, pharmaceutically and legally, with arguments springing up regarding aetiology and risk factors as well. Politically too, they can be contested and there have been well known and large-scale campaigns around individual illnesses, which tend to focus on changing perceptions of a certain disease, altering the tone of education, and improving access to resources, information and infrastructure. A side-effect of these initiatives is that often disenfranchised patients feel like they have been able to recover some dignity and achieve a form of moral reconciliation with a society that has stigmatised and marginalised them. The patient response to the AIDS crisis in the 1980s is almost the epitome of this kind of political contestation, though equally the work of disabled activists, the blind and the deaf movements as well as women's health campaigns could be included here (Epstein, 1996; Lane, 1999).

The way that doctors think we should respond to diseases is another source of conflict. For any given condition there exists a spectrum of medical options. Different treatment programmes are often favoured and promoted across different localities, between individual hospital departments and by doctors themselves, a process which reflects the fragmented, specialised, commercial nature of modern medicine. If alternative remedies are taken into account then it becomes clear that for any condition there exists a plurality of possible medical reactions, not all of which could be considered complementary. Yet this is considered fairly ordinary, and offering patients choice is usually not framed as contestation.

Pharmaceutically, diseases are contested in the sense that a complex and not always symbiotic relationship has emerged in some countries between drug companies, doctors and patients (Elliott, 2011; Goldacre, 2012). I separate this from the clinically arguments discussed above because often this conflict comes to be about more than simply the 'best' way to treat a specific condition. The growth of behavioural disorders, bringing with them fears of over-diagnosis and medicalisation, are a good example of where illnesses become pharmaceutically contested, the arguments being centred around the administration of drugs, the outward pressure on diagnoses, and explaining to some degree both the supply of and demand for treatments (Healy, 2004; Healy, 2012; Lane, 2008).

Related to the sometimes murky clinical and pharmaceutical picture, many diseases could be considered to be aetiologically contested. This terminology is loose, but its basic essence is easy to discern: how exact, numerous and contradictory are our explanatory models? Do different descriptions of potential causality compete in the academic space for legitimacy? It is clear that having a full aetiological picture is no prerequisite for diagnosis, prognosis or treatment. Autoimmune diseases are a case in point of this kind of conflict, as discussions around aetiology remain speculative and varied (Alzabin and Venables, 2012). Even when considering diseases whose mechanism or causes we have known for some time, it should be noted that research is constantly being undertaken to expand our understanding. Many common conditions, whose clinical features have been recognised for centuries, have only relatively recently begun to be understood more fully from an aetiological standpoint and often their histories are ones of treatment before understanding, or indeed treatment on the basis of false understanding (Clarke, 2012).

Legally, diseases have become central to fights over dismissal from work, welfare access and compensation. Employment rights rapidly expanded during the 20th century, and part of this process was the acknowledgment that work environments can make people sick, that sometimes people are too sick to work and that this 'right to be sick' needs to be protected and legislated for (not to say there were not examples from the 19th century: Schivelbusch, 2014). However, given the clear conflict of interest here between the state, employers and the individual, it is inevitable that vigorous and lengthy legal battles will and do ensue. Often what is under scrutiny is the legitimacy of symptoms, the extent to which they disable and the degree to which prognosis of the condition suggests functional limitation.

The reason for this brief exposition of the various ways in which aspects of disease can be contested is to illustrate the simple point that a condition may be disputed in some or even most of the ways above and *still not be considered* a 'contested illness'. There is a further jump that must be taken in order for a disease to become contested, which is hard to precisely quantify, but involves a composite of the above, leading the medical community and society at large to fundamentally doubt the condition in a stronger, more ontological sense. It is this questioning of *being* I have taken to be the hallmark of a contested disease. How can we develop this definition?

A good place to start is to look at the work of Swoboda (2005), who provides the following five points as key features of contested illnesses:[2]

1 Their aetiologies are ambiguous.
2 Their existences are linked to other diagnoses and co-morbid conditions.
3 Their treatment regimens are unclear.
4 Their legal, medical and cultural classifications are disputed.
5 Their statuses as legitimate illnesses are highly controversial.

Taken together, this schema is useful for understanding how a condition comes to be considered contested. What is perhaps unclear is how some

2 I have changed the order for clarity, in the original, number 5 was placed first.

diseases can be said to fulfil numbers 1–4 without necessarily entailing that the fifth condition becomes a feature of the illness. How is it that an illness becomes or is contested in four of the ways mentioned above but does not lose its status as a legitimate illness? And if we establish that the first four criteria are not necessary for describing a contested illness, then how do we avoid tautology in our definitions?[3] In this section I will approach these questions with a mind to revising Swoboda's list to more accurately capture the key components of disputed, or, as I have phrased it, ontologically contested diseases.

To explore this, let us take two examples – asthma and chronic fatigue syndrome (CFS) – and discuss why one is ontologically contested and the other is not with reference to the above formulation. Asthma is chosen here as, superficially, it fulfils much of the criteria above, and yet remains emphatically not a contested disease. CFS is, however, very much considered to be a contested illness, and the following discussion should hopefully clarify why it is rendered such while asthma is not.

Chronic fatigue syndrome versus asthma

CFS presents significant diagnostic and professional challenges for healthcare providers. Patients complain of tiredness, lethargy and dangerously low levels of energy. Cognitive difficulties appear simultaneously; forgetfulness and trouble focusing through to severe migraines and depression. Exercise is painful and can often lead to lengthy recovery periods of forced inactivity and musculoskeletal pain. These symptoms ebb and flow and change day to day, but rarely disappear entirely. There seems to be no abnormality in standard clinical indicators of illness: blood pressure, blood sugar and heart rate don't appear unusual in patient populations, clinical examinations proffer no results, CAT scans likewise. Overall, it is extremely difficult to diagnose CFS in any orthodox manner, and when given it is normally classified as a diagnosis of exclusion, that is, a diagnosis arrived at after other possibilities have been eliminated. The criteria generally used require persisting fatigue for at least 6 months which is not explained by other medical or psychiatric conditions and is not alleviated by rest (Fukuda, 1994; NICE, 2007).

To return to Swoboda's definition, we can note immediately that the aetiology of CFS is unclear. However, the same is true for asthma. Causal models that deal with asthma tend to focus on highlighting prenatal, childhood, environmental and genetic risk factors which include firm links such as maternal smoking, family history and environmental pollution and weak links like exposure to allergens, diet and nutrition, stress levels and breastfeeding (Subbarao, Mandhane and Sears, 2009). All factors are sufficient but not

3 That is, a contested disease being defined by its status as a legitimate disease being highly contested.

necessary, and overall the aetiological picture is stubbornly multifarious; despite a large amount of research over a number of years, it is difficult to discern clearly *what causes asthma*.

Similarly, CFS has no universally accepted aetiology, but rather numerous conceptual models based around physiological, psychosomatic and psychological frameworks (Tveito, 2014). It does differ from asthma however, in the sense that far more moral onus is put on the various causal explanations. The conflicts that exist tend not to be probabilistic discussions about the importance of this or that influence on the condition, but represent a more dogmatic, factional process.[4] Many patients strongly reject all models which identify psychosomatic or psychological factors as primary agents from the conviction that what they are suffering from must be organic. The implication here is that if their condition is not organic then the twin spectres of control and responsibility come into focus: the supposed control of symptoms and the subsequent responsibility for them.

What is different, then, is that to CFS patients, the contested aetiology of their condition has ontological consequences in a way which the causal relationships behind asthma do not. This is because in the case of CFS, the aetiology exists in an explanatory void – it is a conflict about the existence of evidence, rather than what the evidence means. Doctors cannot say with confidence what causes either condition, but with asthma this ignorance is buttressed by various smaller pieces of knowledge: it is like we have most of the puzzle pieces but can't put them together to form the complete image. Determining the aetiology of CFS is a far less certain exercise, and the lack of substantive evidence one way or the other contributes to suspicions that without causal links of some kind we should question whether we are looking at a disease *at all*. From this short comparison it seems that the Swoboda's first condition needs to be modified or expanded to take into account gradations in the types of aetiological ambiguities that are present.

Her second condition – that contested illnesses are linked to other diagnoses and co-morbid conditions – again appears to apply to both asthma and CFS. The former has long been known to be strongly associated with and in some cases exacerbated by many other conditions. In two separate, recent reviews, a high number of comorbid conditions were identified, including rhinitis, gastroesophageal reflux disease, bronchitis, atherosclerotic cardiac disease, psychopathologies and numerous others (Boulet and Boulay, 2011; Ledford and Lockey, 2013). The precise relationship between these conditions is important to clarify as they can often obscure diagnosis and make

4 That is to say, groupings of researchers, activists and patients congeal around different causal explanations, not always on the basis of the best available evidence. Models are often given preference because of their acceptability to the social or psychological prejudices of the person preferring them rather than anything that could be considered scientifically compelling.

treatment more difficult. Establishing links between other diseases and asthma has consequences for patients but also for public health policy.

CFS is also known to have a high comorbidity with other diseases. Fibromyalgia, irritable bowel syndrome, multiple chemical sensitivity, interstitial cystitis and psychiatric conditions such as depression and anxiety disorders have all been found in high prevalence among CFS patients (Aaron et al., 2001; Denise et al., 2012). The way that these conditions interact and influence each other is unknown, and again highly disputed by patients in a way that is unique to contested illnesses. For example, many CFS sufferers would argue that depression is a result of their debilitating fatigue, whereas researchers often posit that this connection is actually the inverse, or that both stem from the same source. Asthma patients do not have such a hostile relationship to their comorbidities.

The crucial point here is that while asthma is associated with mostly 'organic' conditions, CFS finds itself entangled in a web of other contested illnesses or psychiatric diseases. In fact, the one comorbid feature of asthma that is resisted more than any other by patients is the suggestion that there are psychosomatic elements to the disease, hence literature which urges a careful and sensitive approach to the topic (Muramatsu, 2001). Also notable is that the Global Initiative for Asthma (GINA) lists numerous factors which contribute to the development of asthma but only notes that emotional stress and psychiatric conditions can exacerbate the disease (Moes-Wójtowicz et al., 2012). This is in contrast to the ICD-10 (the 10th revision of the World Health Organization's International Statistical Classification of Diseases and Related Health Problems), which places psychological and behavioural causes alongside organic and environmental ones, indicating that there is a slight discrepancy between the medical view and patient outlooks.

So, to look again at the criteria, it seems in this case that expansion of the second point is also necessary. What is important is not so much that comorbidities exist, but the types of connections themselves that the condition has with other diagnoses and the perceived validity of those diseases. Especially relevant here is the question of psychiatric and psychosomatic disorders: if it appears that an illnesses is mostly associated with these types of diseases then I suggest that it will in turn be more likely to be considered contested.

The third feature under discussion here is that in general the treatment regimes of disputed illnesses are unclear. In this case it seems that there is more of a clear dichotomy between my two examples. While the treatment of asthma has certainly changed historically, it is generally accepted that in most cases we can now manage the symptoms effectively in wealthy nations both in acute emergencies and in the long term. There would appear to be very little that is 'contested' about this.

CFS presents far more significant challenges for doctors and patients, as few treatments have been found to have any consistent effect on those with the illness. A plethora of different ideas and potential cures have been suggested, and patients attempt various regimes, largely without success. Responses to treatment are extremely idiosyncratic – what works for one rarely works for another – and those with CFS can grow pessimistic over time as to the effectiveness of any new programme that is suggested to them. Attempts to relieve symptoms such as chronic pain likewise suffer from inconsistent patient response which makes it difficult to draw conclusions across the whole condition.

Two controversial treatments have been fairly widely touted as having therapeutic benefits for CFS patients: cognitive behavioural therapy (CBT) and graded exercise therapy (GET). Part of the justification for using GET is that over time patients' cardiovascular and muscular strength deteriorates due to inactivity, which contributes to maintaining fatigue symptoms. The two methods used in tandem are an attempt to restore physical strength gradually and combat unhelpful views about the disease and the dangers of exercise. These treatments have not been shown to help all patients, but it has been argued that in a significant number of cases they can be effective (Wallman et al., 2004; Whiting et al., 2001; Price et al., 2008).

However, among some patients and a select band of researchers, these approaches are often rejected because they rely on a psychosocial model of illness, or because the design of studies is thought to be flawed. GET has also been argued to cause damage to patients through over-exertion. The flagship paper which promoted its benefits as a treatment regime – known as the PACE trial – has been criticised heavily in what became an ongoing and acrimonious dispute, cumulating (thus far) in an open letter to the *Lancet*, signed by over one hundred academics, patient groups and doctors, calling on the journal to commission an independent reanalysis of the data.

In the case of CFS, simply stating that 'treatment regimes are unclear' misses the most important aspect of this. It is not just that they are unclear, it is that they are inconsistent and, crucially, largely impotent. If we think of a disease like multiple sclerosis (MS), perhaps more suitable for comparison here than asthma, then what we see is a condition that debilitates, destroys, and is ultimately unmanageable in a way that asthma isn't. However, numerous therapeutic interventions exist for MS which can manage symptoms, slow progression and aid recovery from attacks. The precise aetiology of MS remains unknown, but its symptoms *can* be effectively treated, if you allow that treatment doesn't always have to result in the total alleviation of distress or some kind of restoration to pre-disease health. Within the parameters of the disease, we can do more to help those diagnosed with MS than we can for their CFS counterparts and this is I think where treatment contributes to the ontological doubt surrounding the disease.

Swoboda's fourth point is that contested illnesses' legal, medical and cultural classifications are disputed. What she is arguing is that the way the disease is represented, talked about and assumed by many *to be*, exists in constant flux between interested groups. Arguably, this is the case with asthma.

Asthma no doubt intersects the legal system at certain points, though less than many other conditions. It is rare, but not unheard of, for individuals to be discriminated against for their condition, and there have been a smattering of unfair dismissal cases reported in the press. Since asthma is largely a childhood disease, an important way that its legal 'classification' is contested is in relation to healthcare and welfare access, especially under insurance-based healthcare system such as the USA. Making sure that your child can get the care they need is often a legal issue, and links have been established between barriers to access, socio-economic status and mental health of the families involved (Wood et al., 2002). Also in the US, the vast majority of states have passed 'inhaler carry' laws, which entitle students to take prescription medicine on school premises and provide information for educational authorities. The legal classification here is again based around access to resources.

Asthma also features in public health campaigns and attempts to improve workplace and public air safety. This has had success in reducing occupational asthma through the identification and eradication of harmful agents, contributed towards reducing pollution and had an effect on the second-hand smoke debate. Overall however, it would be a stretch to say that asthma is primarily understood legalistically beyond a minority of contexts, and as such its legal classification does not particularly figure as a ground for conflict. The legal work that surrounds asthma is certainly less acrimonious than that for CFS.

As discussed earlier, some medical aspects of asthma are shrouded in ambiguity, and to researchers it is a real aetiological puzzle. But whether or not this actually represents something that can be classified as a dispute is unclear. Asthma is regarded as fairly stable medically in a way that CFS is not, and I think this is the key factor here. Most diseases possess some kind of medical uncertainty, but that uncertainty does not always translate into conflict.

Culturally, it is easy to see how asthma might fit into the schema we are using. The cultural meaning of asthma has been for many years a case of crude stereotyping: asthmatics are routinely typified as the weak, sickly coward, unable to partake in physically or emotionally strenuous exercise without recourse to their trusty inhaler. Clark (2012) carried out a content analysis on 66 Hollywood films and discovered that by far the two biggest standard representations of children with asthma were negative. First, asthmatics were portrayed as socially different in a negative sense (i.e. a misfit of some kind, a nerd or a wimp); and second, asthma is most often a stress response to a situation.[5] It should also be noted that there was a time when others were implicated in the production of asthmatic symptoms, namely

5 A lesser-known archetype for asthma sufferers also exists: that of the individual determined to exert themselves *because* of their asthma rather than *in spite* of it. Che Guevara is one such example of an individual whose condition in part drove him to become more rather than less energetic, as part of a 'stubborn personal battle to beat asthma' (see 'Cuba: Castro's Brain' in *Time Magazine*, August, 1960). As a severely asthmatic child myself, my parents greatly encouraged me to

over-protective, 'smothering' mothers whose concern for their child's health was argued to have become pathological (Appignanesi, 2009).

Looking at CFS, it is clear that it does indeed find its legal, medical and cultural classifications in a state of bitter negotiation. A large portion of the frustration and disappointment felt by CFS and other patients with contested illnesses is related to their perceived lack of legal rights. In areas of employment and welfare, sufferers consistently report finding themselves in the midst of a seemingly contradictory struggle: the struggle to prove themselves fit enough to work in order to stay employed and then the subsequent struggle to prove themselves ill enough to be entitled to state support should the first strategy fail.

Medically, it is difficult to analyse the current view of CFS without making reference to both the fairly wide-spread consensus of the profession that this condition has psychosomatic elements and the equally wide-spread rejection of that consensus by patients. What is different about this kind of conflict is that far greater disagreements exist between patients and doctors than between different researchers, something which is made even more extraordinary when you consider the vague and underdetermined clinical picture.

Cultural wrangling over the meaning of CFS has been explored by Hossenbaccus and White (2013), who carried out a content analysis of medical publications, patient organisation websites and newspaper articles about the condition. They discovered, not to their surprise, a large discrepancy between patient organisations, of whom 89% represented CFS as an organic disease, and medical authorities, who tended to regard it as having both physical and psychological elements (63%). Media outlets were fairly split, 58% portraying it as a wholly physical condition. The imbalance present here gives us clear indicators as to the nature of the cultural dispute. Again it comes back to patients (or patient organisations) being strongly resistant to a psychological label (no matter what form it comes in) and medical researchers reaching for one out of a lack of alternative explanations.

There is another side to this cultural representation too, which is the prevalence of negative perceptions of CFS patients among doctors and wider society. In a recent study examining medical students' views of the disease, common prejudices such as sufferers being 'lazy' or sharing negative personality types, as well as being difficult patients, surfaced regularly among the participants (Stenhoff et al., 2015). Largely, it appeared these views had been absorbed from superiors and media reports. Shorter (1994) suggests that this has always been the case, historically. He writes (ibid., p. 24) that 'knowing they were not facing organic disease, organically oriented physicians tensed up whenever they encountered chronic somatisers' (meaning patients whose bodies subconsciously converted emotional distress into physical symptoms).

swim and play other sports rather than trying to protect me through enforced abstention, so I recognise and appreciate this alternative model of the asthmatic.

Individuals with contested illnesses regularly report that these views are present among family members, friends and work colleagues. Unsurprisingly, patients try to fight these perceptions and wrestle the cultural meaning of their disease towards their advantage.

It should also be noted, perhaps without surprise, that there is not an abundance of positive narratives for the CFS sufferer to mediate their experience through – at least outside of patient-run, sympathetic environments – no survivor or stoic archetype, simply the well-worn clichés of the workshy or the overworked, the hysterical young woman or the hysterical middle-aged one.

Without negating the damage done from such representations and disputes, what I think needs to be made explicit in this discussion is that in large part the legal, medical and cultural classification of CFS emerges from a state of scientific uncertainty. The identity of patients is not stretched and distorted because they belong to a persecuted minority, or because some powerful group has an interest in marginalising how they feel about their disease, it is altered because there is genuine scientific doubt about how to classify, explain and treat it, which in turn interacts with existing social beliefs about illness. This is not the case for asthma, and hence when we look at legal, medical and cultural classifications it is not enough to simply assert that they are in some way conflicted – we need to ask why they are considered in that way and what sustains the dispute.

By way of a short detour, it might be worth considering this discussion in light of research on uncertainty, stemming from the work of Donald MacKenzie and others in the 1990s (MacKenzie, 1990; Wynne, 1992; MacKenzie, 1998). What he showed was that the assumed relationship between expertise and confidence in a knowledge base – that those with the greatest access to information and experience in the field would be the most confident in both the facts of that discipline and the technology it produced – is an over-simplified view and in many cases wrong. Instead of the expected linear relationship, where uncertainty increases the further you get from the site of knowledge production, a different model was proposed whereby those closest to the beating heart of a field are more unsure and reluctant to make strong claims than those from other, neighbouring disciplines. Those who are far away from the production of knowledge but for whom something is at stake could be expected to express the greatest degree of uncertainty.

That is to say that uncertainty exists in the first group, those actually conducting the studies and designing the technology, is minimised or 'black boxed' by the second, those who still work with it but not directly, and emphasised, focused on and potentially exaggerated by those furthest away who have a vested interest in magnifying the appearance of doubt (Latour, 1987; Latour, 1999). Thus it is that those working directly on climate change or the relationship between lung cancer and smoking have a higher degree of suspicion in their causal models than the scientific community as a whole, but less than that which is relentlessly promoted by organisations and individuals who profit from a view of science that is socially constructed and fundamentally uncertain (Oreskes and Conway, 2011; Latour, 2004). This final point, of something *being at stake* for some groups, is key to understanding this argument. In uncontentious areas of science, such ambiguity in knowledge production is less obvious because there is no-one who benefits from doubt. The line goes that climate change modelling on a planet other than Earth would look very different from what we are seeing today, because it would not exist in a social matrix containing organisations strongly invested in maintaining and expanding the infrastructures which contribute to man-made temperature increases.

It gets slightly complicated when we try to apply this to CFS, because we need to be careful not to conflate this certainty/uncertainty axis with the ambiguous/unambiguous scale I have been discussing.[6] That is to say, given that the 'facts' of CFS are themselves so tenebrous, speaking of certainty loses its bite somewhat: it may be that those related to the disease in some way are perfectly certain of its ambiguity across different measures (just as they may be perfectly uncertain of its unambiguity). However, what is useful is the both the idea that there is a three step variance in certainty as you move away from the position of greatest knowledge, and the idea that having something *at stake* is vital in understanding the motivations of those who seek to undermine the level of certainty attributed to a set of beliefs about a concept.

The first of these, the line of uncertainty, does not act in the same way as it appears to in other areas of contentious science. Insofar as you can chart uncertainty stretching from researchers in the field to GPs to patients (the three groups I feel most isomorphic with the general model), certainty levels vary between groups in relation to the supposed fact being discussed, with some drawing divergent responses and some producing a flat line of agreement. This is predictable and explainable. What is of more interest is discussing what effect a vested interest – there being something at stake – might have on the levels of uncertainty.

It would seem, or it seems very much to me, as though the vested interests of all parties involved are in the direction of certainty about the unambiguity of CFS. Medical scientists want to understand what is going on, to be able to model the condition accurately and produce efficacious therapies; doctors want to be able to treat patients, to feel as though they have succeeded in their roles as healers; patients want to comprehend what is going on in their bodies, to be able to communicate that to those around them and, most of all, to get well. All of these groups would therefore benefit from a reduction in the ambiguity of CFS (whether that is framed as uncertainty about unambiguity or certainty about ambiguity) and none of those involved has any interest in promulgating the current view of CFS. But still we remain in a position of fairly widespread doubt as to the solidity of CFS – as a distinct condition, as a condition whose causality we understand, as an illness we can treat

6 Special thanks to Havi Carel for bringing this to my attention.

effectively. It therefore seems fairly convincing to me to posit that the ambiguity here is genuine and does not come about because of any vested interest one way or the other – that is to say the evidence that exists *genuinely* does not provide us with an adequate and reliable explanation for CFS, even to the standard of other (ambiguous but less so) aetiological frameworks.

I hope that this example has not been too exhaustive, but I also hope that it has gone some way to clarifying what makes a disease ontologically disputed. In light of the discussion above, it may be best to conceptualise contested illnesses as lying at the end of a spectrum.

This range encompasses the many diseases that are profoundly manifest in their effects: those that change the colour of our skin, make us cough up blood, kill us, as well as those which are benign and easily coped with; it holds illnesses which we know a lot about and those of which we know very little; it contains conditions that we can treat effectively, and those we cannot, sickness we can clinically observe and that bodily disquiet that evades our gaze.[7] Most diseases are to be found somewhere on this map, between the different axis of effect, understanding and visibility, but contested illnesses lie at the very border, unobserved and unexplained, 'exaggerated cases of biomedicine's inevitable encounter with uncertainty' (Barker, 2005, p. 43).

To summarise, below is a version of Swoboda's original criteria of contested diseases, revised in light of this discussion:

1 Their aetiologies are ambiguous: a solid empirical basis on which to determine between different speculative models is lacking; firm causal processes – mechanistic or probabilistic – are notable by their absence; diagnosis is likely from exclusion.
2 Their existences are linked to other diagnoses and co-morbid conditions: mostly these themselves will struggle with 'legitimacy', they will be psychiatric or psychosomatic in nature, rarely will a clear relationship with an established organic disease exist.
3 Their treatment regimens are unclear; effective treatments are difficult to find: highly inconsistent results are reported among patients.
4 Their legal, medical, and cultural classifications are disputed: there exist discrepancies along these lines between patients and the medical community/society at large; this emerges from genuine scientific doubt and uncertainty, not prejudice.

Therefore:

1 Their statuses as legitimate illnesses are highly controversial and they should be considered ontologically contested diseases.

7 In talking of 'effects' here I am referring to those which can be certified by biomedical apparatus.

Before I bring this chapter to a close and move on to discuss some of the main concepts that orbit disease, it is worth considering for a moment the fact that most ontologically contested illnesses are also chronic, and that this in itself brings a new dimension to the way in which they are experienced but also categorised and received.

Chronic illness

Chronic diseases deserve attention in part because they present huge costs, both human and financial, to health and social systems around the globe, though most notably in the developed world. Essentially, the better doctors become at treating short-term, self-limiting conditions, the more the burden of healthcare transfers to longer-lasting, less curable diseases and the medical emphasis switches from response to management. Already, chronic conditions are estimated to account for up to 70% of deaths in the US and it has been noted that demographic trends, especially in the UK and US, point towards an unbalanced population with disproportionately more older people (who are the main sufferers of chronic illness) than ever before (Thrall, 2005). Thrall notes that 'the magnitude of the population burden of chronic disease is eye-opening' (ibid., p. 10).

The cultural meanings of chronic illness are constantly being renegotiated, and patients often face misunderstandings about the nature of their condition and stigma about their life choices, suffering as they do from diseases which directly contradict that which is valued by our societies – youth, vitality, physical fitness, financial success and general overachievement. I wish to discuss chronic illness here specifically because of the way that chronicity intersects with other features of contested diseases and create layers of conflict both within a patient's environment and themselves. Overriding philosophical ideas – how we view the body and the nature of disease – clash with the lived experience of chronic illnesses and contradict our prior beliefs about disease, even before we have got to some of the exacerbating factors described above.

Arthur Frank (2013), in his excellent book *The Wounded Storyteller*, confronts this dissonance narratively. Frank explains that people tend to talk about their diseases in ways which either conform or confront our expectations of what an ill person should be like. The most common attitude and method of communicating as a sick individual is termed the 'restitution narrative', that is, the story of a person who has recently become ill but is trying to, and will, recover soon. Think, for example, of commonplace 'battle' narratives as they relate to cancer: people win their war with the disease or they lose their brave fight, or else they hang in there while medicine attacks the cancer in a war of attrition, hoping to become survivors. Frank writes (ibid., p. 77) that 'contemporary culture treats health as the normal condition that people ought to have restored. Thus the ill person's own desire for restitution is compounded by the expectation that other people want to hear restitution stories.'

For Frank the central assumption of the sick role is that people take it up in the belief (both of themselves and others) that they will get better – or at least continue to have faith that they will – and it is this understanding of disease which gives restitution stories their power. However, in the case of many chronic illness, these narratives no longer fit, and in the place of restitution we are left with 'chaos': an unending, spasmodic and unordered view of what is happening. This creates its own problems as it rubs uneasily against the form that doctors and others expect a patient to take: 'clinicians cannot entertain chaos because chaos is an implicit critique of the modernist assumptions of clinical work' (Frank, 2013, p. 111). In the end, the sick are left in uncomfortable state where storytelling – the way that they understand what is happening to them and express it to those around them – breaks down entirely, and this collapse is 'compounded by other people's resistances to non-restitution stories of illness' (ibid., p. 191).

The problems often faced by chronically sick people highlight philosophical points about existing models of disease. These conditions frequently fail to fit into conventional understandings of illness and illustrate the futility of both our common narrative responses and of medical intervention (though only if medical intervention's primary aim is to cure, to end).

Clinically, research indicates that large numbers of chronically ill patients are not happy with the care they receive, and that they do not receive enough or the right kind of assistance (Wagner, 1998; Darker et al., 2014). There is also evidence to suggest that when the condition is limiting (i.e. the individual's social, personal and economic activity is restricted by their illness), then this dissatisfaction is greater (Hewitson et al., 2014).

Literature on this topic is regrettably sparse in some areas. While an excellent sociological tradition exists, from Kleinman to Charmaz, characterised by a devotion to compassionate, humane writing, there is a lack of philosophical work on the subject, something both striking and worrying. Many writings attempt to formulate or critique theories of disease in general, and as such touch on chronic illness incidentally, but few regard it as something that might pose unique problems. One exception exists in von Engelhardt (2008), whose work attempts to situate the experience of chronically ill patients in a broader philosophical context. His argument is that chronic disease generates unique stress and puts demands on interpersonal relationships which mean that 'concepts of health and disease require new definitions'. He goes on to say that philosophers are capable of 'producing valuable interpretations of health and disease that [take] the spiritual or cultural nature of human experience into account, [and question] the established positivistic perspective'. It is time, he is saying, to broaden our writings about chronic disease and recognise that though biomedicine is astonishingly successful at keeping people alive, what we often fail to reflect on is 'the quality, or lived experience, of these many lives that have been saved'.

I think that this (von Engelhardt's) point is key: illness is a topic ripe for philosophical reflection, but chronic disease in particular leads us to question our assumptions around sickness and wellbeing, precisely because it is not accommodated as well (or in some cases, at all) by the metaphysical guide ropes we use to understand medical conditions (Carel, 2014). When he says that the concepts of health and disease need new definitions, he is recognising the inadequacy of our current frameworks when it comes to providing insight into certain types of diseases.

Returning to chronic illnesses, it should be noted that they can also be viewed through the lens of social justice. The way that patients are treated raises serious questions about the distribution of resources within health infrastructure, and there is a large amount of evidence suggesting gender bias in the way that patients are treated (Dusenbery, 2018). Economically, those with long-term conditions who suffer the most, outside of their symptoms, are those who are least able to materially support themselves, whether that involves paying for regular medication, hiring carers, modifying their living space or other costs associated with illness. Many are forced to continue working under great bodily distress because the alternative is homelessness and destitution. This is especially apparent in a healthcare system such as the US's, where providing assistance for the chronically ill is not incentivised and therefore underprovided (Walker, 2001). Often the need for more material capital is accompanied by an increased reliance on a social network that can offer help if not always understanding. Thus the weaker a person is connected to others or integrated into such a network at the time of their illness, the more likely they are to struggle with the resulting financial, physical and psychological effects. Havi Carel (2008, p. 74) has written about how the social world of patients, 'so crucial to happiness', can shift and morph as chronic illness wears on. She writes that 'relationships come under new kinds of pressure when the autonomy and independence of the ill person are modified. Old friendships must change to accommodate the illness or eventually wane. New friendships are now formed in the shadow of illness.'

What Carel does not mention in the extract above (though does discuss elsewhere) is how much of this disheartening recalibration of social networks is dependent upon having a strong web of friends and colleagues in the first place, no matter how distressing it is to watch your grip on such relationships loosen or disintegrate. In short, it is those on the fringes of society, those already perhaps marginalised socially and economically from the benefits of living in a developed countries, who find themselves the most worse off should they develop a chronic disease (Marmot et al., 2010).

All of that described above will apply in the majority of cases to individuals with contested diseases – the chaotic illness narratives, the financial struggles, the re-ordering of life around functional concerns – and serves to intersect painfully with the issues that emerge from their specific symptomatic profiles. Patients thus find themselves burdened with the troubles that most chronically ill people face, alongside strange and unaccounted for symptoms. As will be discussed in the next chapter and in the second half of the book, what emerges from the situation is a set of experiences not expected by, nor easily assimilated into, our views of the body and disease, not only from a strictly medical point of view but more broadly. The multitude of ways in which people are ill, in other words, are not fully encapsulated by the modes of thinking we possess to contain them.

Chapter 2

Main concepts

Introduction

What do we talk about when we talk about disease?

The metaphoric dimensions of disease grant it a strange double life as something both grand and personal: racism is a *cancer*, drinking culture a *tumour*; a serial killer's actions – cleaved from the health of the person themselves – are *sick*; but we as individuals are also *ill*, we are *unwell*, we *feel a bit off*; and this is all before we have entered a doctor's office.

It is immediately obvious that I am not discussing disease in terms of *Streptococcus pneumoniae*, or Gleason scores, or mmol/L – that I am talking about a *we* that is non-expert, non-specialised, non-medically trained. This *we* still talks about disease, even if the words are hard to find, the concepts vague, the feelings that need to be conveyed expressed through heuristics and metaphors, buttressed by a technological context and a plurality of supportive reasoning.

The poverty of language in relation to disease, or to the personal expression of disease, is overstated – something I shall return to in my discussion of pain – and as such this chapter will provide an introduction to some of the main concepts that orbit disease, and lay out in consequence a conceptual language with which to make sense of the messy, intractable difficulty of talking about illness. Because we can talk about disease, and we do.

Disease does not arrive alone, conceptually. With it come illness and sickness, legitimacy and validation, responsibility and stigma, all notions that require closer attention if we are to talk about disease. Do these represent discrete conceptual categories, or are they porous and vague? What does it mean to call someone a malingerer, or to be called one? What are we discussing when we speak of biomedicine and the biomedical?

With an understanding of these ideas we possess a language with which to speak of disease – disease-as-lived if not disease-as-treated – and so in this chapter I will try to develop these concepts in a manner that makes clear their interdependence, their shortcomings, their ambiguities and their uses.

Disease, illness, sickness

Talcott Parsons famously wrote in 1951 about the rights and privileges that any ill person could expect to be afforded, providing they conformed with humble enthusiasm to certain anticipated behaviour, namely the 'sick role' (Parsons, 1951). Under his analysis, once one becomes ill it is possible to waive everyday obligations – work, school, being pleasant to others, dressing appropriately – but only in exchange for a demonstrable change in attitude. Isolation is encouraged or in some cases demanded, doctor's orders must be followed and above all a strong will to get better must be ostentatiously displayed. Infantile dependency may be permitted, but solely on the condition that it brings with it an equivalent childlike loss of independence.

The relevance of Parsons's view of sickness-as-deviance to our discussion is not that it states that illness can only exist within the bounds of cultural understanding, a view expressed in a multitude of ways then and since; it is that illness holds no special place in our analysis and can be read as any other social phenomenon – layered with moral implications, certainly, but also an object to be wielded in negotiations with the social world, and one possessed of varying degrees of value to the individual and disturbance to the equilibrium of society as a whole.

Disease is thus a culturally sanctioned and mediated process, and not one that acts upon an individual unknowingly. It need not even be a burden, and may in fact represent a form of escape from a complicated and overwhelming matrix of social responsibilities. Indulging in this form of escapism, surrendering to an invalid tendency, is described by Parsons as a 'tantalisingly attractive "solution"' (Parsons and Fox, 1952, p. 237). It is worth remembering too how much Parsons was influenced by the study of disease and the human body, and that the work of prominent physiologists such as Cannon and Henderson on homeostasis massively informed his ideas about the interrelationship between constituent parts of a social system and its environment.

Parsons's ideas about sickness are now out of fashion, slipping into relative obsolescence due to both the now long-passed turn against functionalism and more substantive social shifts, among them the decline of acute conditions and co-current rise of chronic illness, the refashioning of the doctor-patient relationship – driven in part by the rise of patient advocacy groups and identity movements based around illness – and the pathologisation of normal behaviour (Varul, 2010), but discussion about disease, illness and sickness continue to occupy medical sociology, medical anthropology and the philosophy of medicine.

Since Parsons, who was not concerned with individuated experience, significant gaps have emerged between what may at first appear synonymous terms, and there now in many disciplines exists firm distinctions which split the concept of disease from illness and sickness as they are understood and utilised.

To my mind the best, most lucid articulation of disease, sickness and illness as sociological concepts was written over 40 years ago by Marshall Marinka

(1975). His description to a remarkably full extent captured the way in which these ideas would be used in the years following and are still employed today. He starts with diseases: these are the 'central facts' that inform the medical view, they can be measured, quantified, somehow touched by apparatus and observation. There is a statistical objectivity to them, they present themselves as a 'deviation from a biological norm'. Diseases, then, are discoverable, universal, comparable and consistent.

Illness skirts such neat definition. It is 'a feeling', something inward, only accessible by the patient, an 'underworld of experience'. Illness is a subjective, personal process and entry to it for outsiders is entirely reliant on the ways in which the individual chooses or is able to communicate their experience. Importantly, it is inconsistent and variable. Illness here is fully demarcated from disease, in that there is no obligation that one should follow the other, despite them so often being bedfellows. To be ill but not diseased in the sense outlined here will occupy much space in this work. Not only is illness subjective, but it is also sometimes implied that unlike the other concepts it is something of a personal decision, as Boyd writes, 'whether or not someone is ill, is something the person concerned must ultimately decide for him- or her-self. But whether that person has a disease or is sick is something doctors and others dispute' (Boyd, 2000, p. 11).

Marinka adopts an essentially Parsonsian view of sickness, in that being sick is regarded as a negotiation between a person and society over which liberties can be taken and how favourably or unfavourably their actions will be received. It is a public manifestation, and does not require the presence of either disease or illness as antecedents. Boyd states that 'the security of this role depends on a number of factors, not least the possession of that much treasured gift, the disease'. Still, a person could be regarded as sick by society and adopt the sick role without in fact having any discoverable, biomedical irregularities or indeed feeling unwell subjectively.

As a way of fleshing out these distinctions, let us consider the strange case of Joshua Norton (Lis, 2015). A 19th-century British-American businessman who lost his entire fortune due to an inopportune change in the rice markets, he emerged several years after this calamity to proclaim to the people of San Francisco that he was the 'Emperor of the United States and Protector of Mexico'. Encouraged by the local press and a good-humoured public, he dressed in regal attire and found himself indulged by greetings of mock reverence and 'taxes' wherever he went, despite continuing to live in poverty. Though retrospective diagnosis is a dangerous game, it is not such a stretch of the imagination to believe that had Norton been 'suffering' from that which is most likely – grandiose delusions, a psychiatric disorder with no identifiable organic base – he would have been sick but not ill or diseased. That is to say, he was granted the benefits of sickness on a social level without possessing either a lesion (disease) or indeed consciously experiencing symptoms (illness).

Following Marinka, Arthur Kleinman (1988) added his voice to the discussion and strove for a more detailed though similar description of disease and illness, alongside an expanded and reconceptualised vision of what sickness might mean. In his view, sickness incorporates all the macro-social elements of disorders, be it economic, class, gender, racial or institutional factors. Poor housing, job pressures, family life; all of these, for Kleinman, became elements of sickness that were previously ignored. His explicit desire in separating the three was to highlight the ways in which illness and sickness were ignored by a medical community overly focused on curing disease, and the lack of compassion, bad practice and poor public policy that resulted.

Since the work of these authors many subtle variations have emerged but most retain the basic distinction that disease is something biomedical, illness is something personal and sickness is something societal. An indicator of this continuity can be found in Aho and Aho's 2008 work *Body Matters: A Phenomenology of Sickness, Disease, and Illness*, where they write that disease is 'an organic pathology as discerned by one or more recognised clinical or laboratory procedures' and illness is 'a non-quantifiable lived experience, not feeling well' (Aho and Aho, 2008, p. 3). Later in the same text (ibid., p. 77) they sum up by stating 'physical and mental troubles show up in society as sickness-deviations to be corrected. To patients, they disclose themselves as illnesses. To doctors, ailments present themselves as diseases to be cured.' This view is virtually indistinguishable from that presented three and a half decades previously by Marinka. Further evidence of the entrenchment of these conceptual boundaries can be found in other places. Wikman et al.'s (2005) study, for example, attempted to operationalise disease, sickness and illness along these now-familiar lines. Professionally diagnosed conditions stood in for 'disease', self-reported bad health was used for 'illness' and 'sickness' was represented by absence from work on sick-leave.

Although some theorists departed from Marinka's basic view, the essential features of their schema have remained unusually stable as sociological concepts. Such is the influence of their work that the idea of disease as 'objective', illness as 'subjective' and sickness as 'macro' or 'societal' is now in fairly common usage across not just sociology but also medical anthropology and the philosophy of medicine. Disputes occur, but generally these take place within the predetermined boundaries described above rather than around the actual ontological validity of such distinctions (for example, see Twaddle and Nordenfelt, 1993, or Hofmann, 2002).

Given its longevity, this approach evidently has an enduring appeal to theorists. Indeed, it seems to fairly intuitively capture what are closely related and overlapping but distinct concepts. There is a sense of validity about the idea that a disease is an individual, measurable, pathological entity or dysfunction which (in most cases) *causes* you to feel ill, the precise sensation of which, mediated by cultural context and personal interpretation, represents illness, followed by a phone call with the boss and chicken noodle soup from your partner (i.e. the social benefits of sickness), but that these three concepts follow on from, interact with and are closely related to each other without being exactly the same thing.

No doubt, too, for a theorist working to challenge a biomedical system that has obvious downsides for patients suffering from some conditions, the creation and assertion of these distinctions allows a shift in focus away from primarily reductionist medical concerns and a proclamation that the subjective and the societal matter. As such, Cecil Helman wrote in 1988 that splitting disease and illness 'has been one of the most useful contributions of medical anthropology' and as recently as 2016 Havi Carel has asserted the desirability of separating them (Helman, 1988; Carel, 2016c).

This dichotomy is not without issues, however. While it is often stated that disease, illness and sickness are overlapping terms, it is clear to me that there is a hierarchy implicit in their formulation which elevates disease, in all its measurability and delineation, above illness and sickness. As will become evident as we move on to the main topic of this work, to live with a condition such as fibromyalgia or chronic fatigue syndrome is to be ill without disease, and the problems that emerge from such a situation are manifold. I take issue with philosophers who recognise this danger but discount it, such as Carel when she writes:

> [The disease/illness dichotomy] does not imply that illness that is not accompanied by disease is less real or less significant than an illness that is. Indeed, our ability to identify disease is contingent and changes over time. Hence I am not suggesting that an illness that is not accompanied by disease is less real but merely that we have not (yet) identified the disease. The epistemic restriction, namely our current inability to identify the disease, should not drive any ontological assumptions about the reality or severity of the illness.
>
> (Carel, 2016c, p. 587)

My contention with passages such as the above is that they name the problem without addressing it: our current inability to identify disease in some cases *does* drive ontological assumptions about the reality or severity of illness, whether we like it or not, and putting the issue to one side with an assertion of future identification of pathology assumes that all illness can and will one day be explained biomedically, a piece of reasoning that loops back on itself when we wonder why patients with non-identifiable conditions struggle to be taken seriously.

Furthermore, some of the best work in the sociology of science in the second half of the twentieth century was that which unpacked not the exploitative fringe of science but its effective, prestigious core.[1] Maintaining a strict disease/illness distinction brackets disease as the preserve of science, implicitly removing our

1 I am thinking not only of Bloor's Strong Programme and the work of Latour (who, despite their differences, both believe the scientific production of knowledge is ripe for critical analysis), but also of more recent work such as Douglas (2009).

analytic hands from what we know in many cases to be a highly politicised process of definition, fraught with pharmaceutical industry interference, ascendant patient advocacy movements, and long-standing issues of sexism and racism in clinical trials. The danger is that we rob ourselves of the conceptual tools to challenge a set of institutionalised beliefs that we split illness from disease to combat in the first place. As Mansbridge (2001) writes:

> Inequalities in power have their most insidious effect when the dominant group has so much control over the idea available to other members of the society that the conceptual categories required to challenge the status quo hardly exist. Ideological hegemony of this sort pervades every human society in ways that are, by definition, hard to bring to conscious awareness.
>
> (Mansbridge, 2001, p. 4)

Or Kitwood:

> The discourse generated by medical science is so dominant, and supported by such power and prestige, that its anomalies, self-contradictions and non-sequiturs are obscured from view.
>
> (Kitwood, 2002, p. 142)

In this work, then, though I acknowledge the intentions of splitting disease, illness and sickness, I will try and treat the phenomena they signify as coagulated rather than separate – different parts of the same messy thing, a bodily disquiet that oscillates within the junctures of society, biology and subjective experience. Annemarie Mol (2003) talks about meaning-making in disease as a collaborative process between doctor and patient to give shape to the reality of symptoms and their pathological (or otherwise) origins, and this is closest to my position. Maintaining the firm conceptual categories above has outlived its usefulness and, as we shall see, struggles to contribute to our understanding of those whose disease we must take on trust, whose illness is denigrated on the basis of its ill-ability to fit within the structures of legitimacy we have established.

Malingering, validity and legitimacy

Patients with contested illnesses often face accusations of insincerity, of faking or exaggerating symptoms for gain and of being malingerers. It can be unclear exactly what this entails conceptually. What is not unclear is that as a result they feel like their experience is invalidated and their disease is considered illegitimate. In this section we will look at what these concepts mean and how they intersect with those ideas previously discussed.

Let us start with malingering. This is a well-known concept which appears throughout history, but finding actual legal or clinical applications is difficult.

Indeed, though malingering frequents legal, medical and psychiatric spheres it fails to make a home in any of them (Raine, 2003), leaving it best described as an unstable and untested theoretical concept, one that is either subsumed into other categories like fraud or else partially medicalised. However, malingering does carry with it a significant amount of social weight, and examples are easily found in films, books and real-life. This has generated a pejorative set of meanings around the idea, which in turn negatively affect those tarred with its brush.

The basic concept is common knowledge: malingering is the act of pretending to be sick, or of injuring yourself, in order to gain in some way. Although associated firmly with military service, it morphed during the 20th century and expanded, becoming more than just self-inflicted injuries and faked symptoms as ways of avoiding war (Palmer, 2003). Now, it applies to anyone who declares themselves sick, or artificially induces illness in order to gain materially or by being able to give up responsibilities (i.e. to individuals cheating their way into the sick role, without possessing that which is considered an essential quality of membership, namely to be actually ill).

Central to malingering is 'secondary gain', which is the idea that an individual must aim to benefit in some way from their deception. In a 21st-century context, this will ordinarily come in the form of social security benefits, litigation payment or time off work. Emotional rewards are not normally included here, but the sympathy and good-will of others could be added to the overall package of benefits one hopes to achieve through their actions. Malingering stretches from phoning in sick when you are in fact planning to spend the day at the zoo to a calculated deception intended to bring you large rewards, for example pretending to be grossly injured following a workplace accident. Key to this idea is conscious intent: the person involved must be aware of the reasons behind their actions (even if this turns out to be rationalised in an overly simplistic manner or is reliant on false premises). However, secondary gain is a 'highly speculative and empirically untested' concept, and finding medical or legal applications for malingering proves troublesome (Rogers and Neumann, 2003).

Clinically, it can be difficult to recognise individuals who are faking symptoms, and malingering is 'a description of behaviour', *not* a medical diagnosis (Boon et al., 2006). Doctors are not trained or especially expected to identify patients who are deceiving them, and it has been suggested that some 'maintain an undiscerning naïveté' about the potential for patients to lie or deceive (Cunnien, 1997). Malingerers pose a unique problem for doctors in that they invert completely what might be ideally expected from a patient. By 'their very nature' these individuals attempt to 'evade any normal doctor-patient relationship' and enter the surgery or hospital with very different priorities to most (Bayliss, 1984, p. 583). In any case, demarcating this phenomenon from actual disease is a process fraught with difficulty, and clinical skills are not always sufficient for this task. Even equipped with tools such as Symptom

Validity Testing, attributing specific, motivated intent is speculative and malingering remains a 'weak diagnosis of exclusion' (Pankratz and Erickson, 1990, p. 383). Doctors are also not best placed ethically to identify malingerers, and if the levels of fraud reported by the health insurance industry are correct, they are not very successful at it either. This has been partially confirmed by studies which show doctors have difficulty detecting deception in a clinical setting (Jung and Reidenberg, 2007). Ultimately, the case has been put that, as a doctor, in most instances it is more important to accept complaints and symptomatic patterns that you are uncertain of than risk rejecting or belittling genuine distress (Robinson, 2003).

A distinct (though related) concept complicates the clinical picture of malingering. Known as factitious disorders (sometimes referred to as Munchausen's syndrome), they are a family of psychiatric conditions in which patients fabricates illness, either through inducing symptoms or self-reporting problems they don't have. They do this because they want medical attention, whether that comes in the shape of puzzled concern from their doctor, blood tests from the hospital or, in extreme cases, invasive surgery (Folks, 1995).

The aim here is not material gain, and this is what separates it from malingering. Instead, individuals hope to satisfy a psychological need, to allay some deep personal unease through becoming a patient. The lengths to which people will go to get their sick role legitimised are frequently extraordinary, and it is this lack of rational 'cost-benefit' analysis which further distinguishes them from malingerers. The pertinent questions in these cases often becomes: at what point do we consider lying and deceit pathological and does it matter that the gains achieved are not material? In recent times the amount of clinical information available online has widened the opportunities for those with this condition.

Another set of illnesses often confused and conflated with malingering are known as somatic symptom disorders. Though comprising many parts, these largely arise when psychological distress and anxiety in a patient subconsciously transfers or 'converts' into physical symptoms. These manifestations can look and feel no different to the individual than if they were experiencing them in an orthodox manner. Unsurprisingly, somatic symptom disorders have a long and troubled history of confusing and upsetting both patients and doctors. What separates them from malingering is intent: these symptoms are not produced or reported with any desire to deceive, and often doctors have a better grasp of their production than the patient does. There is some common ground between malingering, factitious disorders and somatic symptom disorders, for example the responsibility placed on certain arbiters (normally medical staff) to ascertain the level of conscious awareness that a patient has and their potential motivations (for a more thorough overview, see Bass and Halligan, 2014). Teasing apart these separate but overlapping concepts is not an easy task.

Legally, malingering is a murky and ill-defined entity, and many doubt its existence as a distinct legal concept: Jones (2003) argues that 'malingering is occasionally central but often marginal, if not irrelevant, to the court's decision making process' and Sprince (2003, p. 241) writes: 'the law's position on malingering is characterised by the absence of substantive and definitive features and by an indifference to any imperative to acquire them'. This is largely because it is either captured by existing legal categories like fraud and perjury or lives a life of its own within military and prison structures (where it has a long history).

In specific contexts it does appear to gain a little clarity and distinction: most notably in matters of compensation and welfare. There is evidence of patients faking or exaggerating symptoms in cases of post-traumatic stress disorder, brain injuries, whiplash and chronic pain among others (Rosen and Taylor, 2007; Greiffenstein and Baker, 2005; Greve et al., 2009).[2] However, here the definition of malingering becomes extremely context-dependent, and ambiguities remain, especially surrounding methods of detection. Exaggeration of non-specific symptoms for example can be extremely difficult to prove, and whether it warrants the use of problematic and intrusive methods such as surveillance and character assessment is undecided. Too much weight is put on conjecture to allow malingering to be considered a solid theoretical entity in this situation.

Compounding these problems is the dearth of data that has been collected on malingerers. We have only very rough figures for how many there might be under any given diagnosis, and what this translates into in terms of cost to the healthcare and insurance industries is equally unknown. First-person accounts are lacking for obvious reasons. Malingering is best characterised as a slippery concept that is not fit for purpose in the majority of circumstances that it might reasonably be applied in. Sharpe succinctly describes the difficulties faced by researchers as the following:

> Theoretically, malingering is distinguished from psychiatric illness by the absence of psychopathology, the identification of 'secondary gain', and a conscious intent to deceive in order to obtain the gain. However, psychopathology is hypothetical, secondary gain is non-specific, and the determination of the extent that intent is conscious probably impossible.
>
> (Sharpe, 2003, p. 156)

That is to say, each constituent conceptual part of malingering begins to look suspect under further examination.

This being true, malingering does cast a shadow over our cultural life, and it is here that perhaps it exists most vividly. Malingering is imbued with moral significance, and the osmosis of common tropes by both medical and non-

2 A recent example of this kind of behaviour is the spate of food-poisoning cases brought by British tourists against continental resorts, vastly out of proportion to the other nationalities that holiday there.

medical figures contributes greatly to patients' understanding and experience of the term.

There is no shortage of cultural examples to choose from. Norman Mailer's debut novel *The Naked and the Dead* included a character who attempted to fake the symptoms of nervous shock to get removed from the front-line. *Seinfeld*'s George Constanza pretended to be disabled so that he could access the executive bathroom. The traditional reading of *Hamlet* has the woebegone prince feign (rather than suffer from) madness in order to extract his revenge on Claudius.

Kuperman's (2006) content analysis on representations of malingering in works of fiction identified one consistency that should be noted: 'in fiction, as in the clinic, malingerers often prefer mental disorders to somatic diseases'. Because the majority of mental illnesses are symptomatic – that is, defined only by the symptoms as subjectively reported and recorded – it is a truism that faking such a condition is far easier than altering your body so that it falls in line with the biological indicators of specific conditions enough to trick doctors. It is also a truism that you are more likely to be suspected of malingering if your complaints are symptomatic.

Not to say that there are no non-fictional examples of medical fakery. Consider the extraordinary case of Steven Jay Russell. Among the duplicity and many daring escapes that littered his criminal career, one particular scheme stands out as a masterclass in malingering. Though incarcerated, he was able, through a combination of laxatives, starvation and convincing acting, to fake the symptoms of late-stage AIDS and get himself removed from prison and placed in a hospice (where he subsequently engaged in further ingenious deception and faked his own death in order to escape). Real-life malingerers are not always as eye-catching or inventive as Russell, but they certainly exist.

So, whatever the ambiguity that pervades the theoretical debate around malingering, it is an idea that should not be dismissed. However defined, faking illness, or being thought to fake illness, is an issue which has been growing in importance over the last century and may continue to do so. A troubling trend forms part of the background to this. Since the 1970s, more generous sickness benefits have generally become available across the majority of Western nations. Over the same period, the uptake of such benefits has increased dramatically and without signs of slowing, despite widespread improvements in general levels of public health, occupational safety, dietary information and interventionist medical care. Partially this paradox can be explained by the explosion in the number of 'medically unexplained symptoms' or 'subjective health complaints', which cover the majority of contested illnesses and whose patient populations often attempt to access sickness benefits of one kind or another, but to an extent this phenomenon is underdetermined (Ford, 1997; Binder and Campbell, 2004). In the shadow of this trend lies the suspicion among many that a large number of people are either not sick or not as sick as they say they are.

For many individuals, particularly the ill themselves, the word 'malingerer' is heavily loaded. It represents a host of accusatory connotations which grate against the dominant positive narratives of selfhood present in modern society. To be a malingerer is to be an individual who rejects through their actions the idea that everyone has an obligation to contribute, most often quantified economically, to society. Those who can contribute but who choose not to, or who find ingenious ways of circumventing their responsibility, are allocated to an unsavoury category of individuals, the 'scroungers' and 'cheats' of tabloid headlines. Malingering is thus easily incorporated into a world-view that constructs society out of the worthy – those working in legitimate jobs, living within the law, etc. – who deserve the rewards they receive, and the deceiving underbelly, those who freeload on an overgenerous state. To be a malingerer is by definition to be a liar, and the maintenance of dishonesty more often than not requires a level of devious manipulation not thought to be a positive character trait. People do not accommodate such views of themselves easily, and so it is unsurprising that being regarded in this way often provokes a violent defensiveness.

For patients with contested illnesses, being accused of malingering is a particular concern because of the 'subjective' nature of their complaints. Having a purely symptomatic illness can generate the uncomfortable feeling that those around you and those professionally responsible for your wellbeing have ceased to trust the way that you represent yourself. This is not paranoia: focusing on fibromyalgia for instance, different research has shown that a significant percentage of doctors and a lower but still relevant number of specialists doubt the credibility of the disease, and many believe outright that those who claim to suffer from it are malingering (Hayes et al., 2010; Album and Westin, 2008). What has also been highlighted, as suggested above, is the fairly straightforward way in which the clinical features of the illness could be feigned, and critics point towards the inconsistent reporting of symptoms as further evidence (Johnson-Greene, Brooks and Ference, 2013).

Outright, straightforward, perfectly-well-but-pretending-otherwise cases of malingering are suspected to be relatively rare, however. What is more commonly suggested – and a more interesting process to consider – is that individuals do not feel completely healthy, but that in representing their symptoms they are prone to exaggeration, unnecessary fixation and anxiety, facilitated perhaps by 'an unconscious need to seek legitimisation of symptoms in the context of "disbelief" by others' (Harth and Nielson, 2014). This 'context of disbelief' can be seen through the strategies patients adopt: a morgellons disease organisation, for example, provides a cover letter to show to your physician while other groups emphasise different tactics that will make navigating the benefits system easier. The idea here is not to cheat or deceive, but rather to recognise the often prejudicial circumstances that ill people find themselves in and to make the most of the tools available.

A concept that is sometimes brought into play when discussing these conditions is known as 'compensation neurosis'. This is a term which is often used pejoratively to describe the apparent increase in symptom severity noted in those pursuing compensation which then abides or dissipates following a successful outcome. It has been speculated on this basis that the rise of welfare opportunities for the ill has caused the growth in symptomatic conditions, and that 'financial reward or compensation for self reported pain or suffering would seem to be more harmful than helpful' (Bellamy, 1997, p. 94).

Compensation neurosis is a more complex phenomenon than it first appears: it is not simply a case of individuals overplaying their hand in order to squeeze money out of the system. As Hall and Hall (2012) have argued, finding yourself in a compensatory struggle presents a unique set of stressors, only one of which is potential financial reward. What may be more pertinent is the pressure exerted by lawyers, family and friends to experience your condition in a certain way, or the effect of continually retelling and reasserting your subjective symptoms in a climate of doubt. It is these processes which can in some people (different groups of individuals have been shown to be more or less susceptible) generate the unconscious expansion of symptoms.

As we shall discuss later in this book, there is some truth to the idea that for patients with contested illnesses, symptoms do apparently oscillate in severity over time and across situations. However, this does not appear to me to be a case of patient's exaggerating symptoms in order to gain some kind of reward. Rather, it is two processes occurring simultaneously. The first is the tailoring of disease, or how disease is reported, to the requirement of different contexts. Patients often try to present their condition as much as possible in ways which accord with institutional and societal expectations, most having learnt the hard way that telling the 'truth' (as they saw and felt it) about what they were experiencing was not always fruitful.

The second process at play here is harder to articulate: I have in mind the subconscious effects of living with a symptomatic profile not understood or given meaning within the social matrix of your life, i.e. the struggle to live well and trust your body while lacking empathy and validation from both others around you and the higher-level, intellectual structures we situate our experiences within. Though the effects of this process are hard to define, and fluctuate from individual to individual, it seems clear to me that without the patient's explicit determination, the circumstances they find themselves in may contribute in some instances to a 'hardening' of the way in which they interpret their distress, or indeed the way their body does on their behalf. That being said, for many patients, as I will discuss later on, this persistent retelling and negotiation of their sickness identity appears to generate self-doubt and foster concealment strategies rather than any hardening of symptom narratives. Potentially shorter-term, more one-off compensatory situations, such as those regarding whiplash following an accident for example, seem more likely candidates for compensation neurosis.

Indeed, patients with contested illnesses do occasionally come under bureaucratic scrutiny, but in many instances the hope of financial compensation from the very beginning is understood to be slight, and some do not engage in the process at all. There also seems to be little evidence of patients recovering or part recovering after receiving welfare approval, though it is argued that in the case of chronic conditions these payments incentivise patients to remain ill rather than get better and lose entitlement. In many cases, people remain ill, housebound and unable to work regardless of the level of assistance they receive.

There is one extra component here, touched upon earlier: the incredibly strong and emotive link that people draw between a condition being 'psychological' or 'psychosomatic' and it being under their control. Indeed, patients themselves have been shown to view psychosomatic illness and malingering as synonymous, regardless of attitudes within medicine and psychiatry (Wessely and Showalter, 1999). It is clear that the most important aspect of malingering for those with contested illnesses is *agency*. Agency brings with it that which is dreaded: responsibility. As Hacking (2002, p. 11) states: 'Responsibility is the crux. We have a profoundly moral attitude to disease. If something is a real disease, you are not responsible for it.'

And thus, for some people with contested illnesses, the mere suggestion that *any* part of what they suffer from might be psychological in origin can entail the subsequent conclusion that the person making that diagnosis is accusing them of being in control of their symptoms. That is, since psychosomatic conditions are not 'real' in the eyes of suffers – organic, biomedical conditions being the only ones which 'count' – they are therefore the fault of the individual who contracts them or displays their symptoms. Kirmayer (1988) describes the diagnosis of a psychosomatic condition as transforming the 'real into the imaginary, the innocent into the culpable'. As we shall see in the second half of this book, not all patients reject this label as strongly as is often suggested, some fully incorporating a psychological element to their personal conceptualisation of their condition, but what does remain constant is the desire above all to be absolved of blame. Showalter (1997) writes about why CFS patients prioritise biological explanations by placing them within a broader social context that is sceptical of the 'reality' of non-biological diseases:

> Patients with chronic fatigue live in a culture that still looks down on psychogenic illness, that does not recognise or respect its reality. The self-esteem of the patient depends on having the physiological nature of the disease accepted: the culture forces people to deny the psychological, circumstantial, or emotional sources of their symptoms and to insist that they must be biological and beyond their control in order for them to view themselves as legitimately ill.
>
> (Showalter, 1997, p. 117)

The last two words used above are those that patients most often repeat: their condition is not regarded as legitimate and therefore they are not believed to be legitimately ill. Legitimacy here also means that an ill person *has the right* to feel the way they do, to be excused from working, to receive welfare payments, to expect sympathy, etc. because their condition is 'real'. As a reaction to this, what has been observed across many contested illnesses is the formation of alternative models of legitimation, which posit versions of aetiology, diagnosis, prognosis and treatment that are removed from and sometimes in conflict with the mainstream medical view (Swoboda, 2006). These explanations extend to covering the difficulties that their conditions present and 'helps sufferers deal with conflicting medical and cultural representations of their illnesses by explaining why contested illnesses are so hard to diagnose and treat' (ibid., p. 245).

Closely related to this is the idea of validity: that if a disease is not legitimate then therefore the symptoms and associated distress of the ill person becomes invalid. This is viewed by many patients as a deeply painful denial of their personal experience, especially as it can come not only from medical professionals but from those closest to them – friends, children, partners. A recurring theme among patients with contested illnesses is that although others 'try to understand', nobody except fellow patients really has access to their symptomatic world. A lot of people within the community point to explanatory strategies such as 'spoon theory' as a way of conveying functionally to those without the condition what it is like to suffer from it.[3]

This does not, however, alter the fact that for many patients, the way that their body makes them feel is sufficiently removed from how others perceive that experience as to create severe psychological tension. Despite the attempts of the patient community to pursue alternative legitimatising models and even in possession of fortitude and self-belief, patients still remain engaged in a struggle to validate their embodied existence.

This issue is, I believe, best explained as a form of conceptual distance, whereby the phenomenology of disease for those with contested illnesses (and others) is mismatched with prevailing notions of what disease *should* be, creating a gap between people's expectations and a patient's experience. To begin to look more in-depth at this problem, we must first examine the pervasive but fuzzy historical and philosophical idea, 'biomedicine'.

It is this loose system of thought or, rather, way of seeing and encountering disease, which more than any other set of ideas guides us, both as specialists

3 'Spoon theory' is an analogy that describes the way conducting seemingly mundane and everyday tasks can drain the energy of someone with certain illnesses. People with said illnesses start each morning with a predetermined number of 'spoons', and use them up throughout the day on whatever activities they attempt, to the point where if all spoons are depleted then they have no option but to rest. This is contrasted to able-bodied, healthy people who have a 'never-ending' supply of spoons and do not have to adjust their actions on the basis of how many they have left. This explanatory tool is not used exclusively by people with contested illnesses, but also by individuals with disabilities and other chronic diseases. Kristin K. Barker (2005) describes strategies such as these as *the economy of the body*.

and non-specialists, when it comes to sickness. Though it has brought us many benefits, there are plenty of instances where the biomedical worldview is simply unable to adequately account for phenomena it is expected to assimilate. Contested illnesses being one such group, in which disease experiences are rendered almost entirely incomprehensible by biomedical attempts to classify and explain. Such is the ubiquity of its basic tenets that they have come to represent the common-sense underpinnings of categories like 'disease', and those conditions that do not appear to fit have become strange category errors, unable to ascend to full disease status.[4] The damage done by this incompatibility will be explained at length in Part II of this book. But first, what exactly do we mean when we talk of 'biomedicine'?

Biomedicine

In 1936, Henry Sigerist wrote that 'medicine is not a branch of science and it never will be'. He was engaged in a dispute with George Sarton about the nature of their disciplines' relationship (history of medicine and history of science respectively) at the time, but what is relevant is the way in which he regarded medicine as an intrinsically *social* enterprise. This assertion has not lost relevance. If anything, the need to emphasise those aspects of medicine which are not scientific, especially in relation to the topic at hand here, is greater than in Sigerist's era. This is because of the dominance of the 'scientific' branch of medical practice, which has expanded vastly in scope and power following the Second World War. In this section, I will outline what are regarded as the core features of biomedicine and discuss some common objections and critiques, mostly drawn from sociology. I will then look at the implications of the biomedical model for contested illnesses and bring greater clarity to the notion that this can be framed as a philosophical problem as well as a sociological one.

Though it is possible to trace the beginnings of biomedicine, philosophically, back into the nineteenth century and beyond, through the work of Pasteur, Koch and Bernard (not to mention Broussais, Bichat and perhaps even further to Descartes), it is not an unreasonable assertion to make that the modern features of this phenomenon only began to solidify and permeate in the post-war period, where biological science and clinical practice converged at the start of the antibiotic age (Keating and Cambrosio, 2003). This is because, alongside the new focus on identifying and eliminating foreign agents as a primary method of fighting disease came a new set of assumptions about what medicine *is* and *does*. It is here that a closer, more intimate relationship developed between the laboratory and the hospital, training began to contain an explicit, scientific core and a series of seemingly incredible

4 Though it must be said that contested illnesses, for a variety of reasons, have rarely been fully accepted as completely legitimate disease entities.

victories over long-standing scourges (tuberculosis and syphilis for example) shaped the narrative of interventionist, miraculous medicine (Quirke and Gaudillière, 2008), and it is here that medicine fused itself to the biological sciences once and for all.

Thus it was that a way of seeing the medical world which had long been intellectualised – the development of the dichotomised body as object and subject, the preference for measurement over speech, the invasive technologisation of diagnostic procedures, a general adoption of the principles and methods of biology – spread gradually across the medical and then social worlds of the west, normalised and perpetuated through schools and universities, slowly absorbed by populaces, increment by increment becoming the expected norm (Mol and Law, 2007). Biomedicine has been for some time the dominant viewpoint from which to understand disease, both by many if not all medical personnel and by lay populations, albeit in a much more intangible, fluid manner. But what are its constituent parts? – what do we mean by *biomedicine*?

The core tenets of biomedicine

A good place to start is with Nettleton's (2006) description, which identifies five core tenets, encompassing the major trends without necessitating too much deviation or lengthy exposition. They are as follows:

1 Mind–body dualism: the mind and the body are treated separately; disease relates to the body.
2 Mechanical metaphor: the body is best understood as a complicated machine with independent parts and systems that can be repaired individually.
3 Technological imperative: technological interventions are prioritised; there is a bias towards curing rather than caring.
4 Reductionism: health and illness are explained in strictly biological terms; sociological, environmental or psychological factors are downplayed or disregarded unless no organic cause can be identified.
5 Doctrine of specific aetiology: disease entities are solely responsible for disease.

Mind–body dualism in this context refers to the dichotomy between what are regarded as 'subjective', mental complaints and 'objective', physical ailments, with the latter prioritised as more legitimate. The physical and mental domains of health as schematised here are separated to a large extent in training, research and clinical practice in western medicine. Distinct institutional and professional divisions exist, and generally speaking 'physical' medicine is held in higher esteem – both by the medical establishment and lay persons. This split no doubt contributes to the lack of parity that exists between mental and physical disorders, and the result is often that conditions that do not produce consistent or convincing biomedical markers are more likely to be regarded as suspicious, irrelevant or overly time-consuming by practitioners and as potentially false by non-professionals (Crowley-Matoka, 2009).

The second factor that Nettleton identifies is the employment of a mechanical metaphor to explain how the human body works and by extension how to fix it when things go wrong. Abstract representations of anatomy and physiology include numerous references to the body-as-machine, and medical textbooks regularly and explicitly make this connection. Understanding this is vital to comprehending biomedicine. Foucault (1996), Starr (1982), and others like Bishop link this conception with the history of pathological anatomy and the construction of a normative body from a dead one; the corpse, invaded and manipulated by the dissector's scalpel and electrodes, stands in for the living one, and the patient 'who was the absolute subject of the disease, [becomes] the object against which both the gaze and the analytic probing of the doctor are directed' (Bishop, 2011, p. 55). Over time, they argued, the asymmetry between the power of the physicians gaze – aided by deeper theoretical knowledge and actual technology – and the descriptive tools possessed by patients grew to the point that virtually all of the interpretive burden of the doctor patient encounter fell on the side of medicine, and we ended up where we are today, the body of the patient de-individualised, the perception of embodied distress relegated beneath the various models and tests and pieces of diagnostic equipment that represent the probing fingers of modern medicine.

This process is intertwined with the third and fourth factors: a body that is a machine is an item of interest reduced to a collection of co-existing parts and systems that break down and can be repaired in the same way that complicated mechanical structures are, with targeted interventions aimed at rectifying specific faults. The ambition of biomedicine here is always restoration, and, since natural biological function is considered entirely synonymous with mechanical function, mechanical intervention is likewise the obligatory response. This vein of biomedicine runs deep – the descriptive language we use, the measures we employ to denote success, the way in which studies are designed – and the outcome is well documented. Clinical focus turns to biological rather than psychological or social factors to explain disease, but also, and more crucially here, to *encounter* it. Under biomedicine, health becomes a largely physiochemical concept, quantified statistically, and disease, for many patients, assumes an isolated cause-and-effect dynamic (Helman, 1988). This exemplary materialism creates a world in which 'real' illness 'corresponds to the degree to which physical traces show up in the body … health and illness are defined in terms of materialist indicators' (Gordon, 1988, p. 24).

The central tension here is perhaps best explicated by Canguilhem when he writes:

> The living organism acts in accordance with empiricism, whereas the machine, which is the product of calculation, verifies the norms of

> calculation, that is, the rational norms of identity, consistency, and predictability. Life, by contrast, is experience, that is to say, improvisation, the utilisation of occurrences; it is an attempt in all directions.
>
> (Canguilhem, 2008, p. 90)

Precisely this – the *attempt in all directions* – is what separates life as it is lived and life as it is constrained by biomedicine; the diseases we will discuss in this book are unassimilated into existing biomedical categories and perhaps will remain so, and yet the force of their empirical effects is indisputable. The reconciliation of these two processes is a major theme of this work, but it also a major theme of many people's lives, and the constant friction between what they feel and what they believe to be true, or what those around them believe to be true, can be isolating and confusing, and profoundly damaging to the integrity of a patient's identity. As Bishop writes:

> Sometimes we cannot recognise things about ourselves. We so inhabit our dogmas (or shall I say, our dogmas so inhabit us?) that to question our beliefs – those things that our time and our society have taught us to be true and good, and indeed beautiful – threatens who we are. We cannot see who or what we have become, because what we have become does not appear for us, does not make itself known, even while what we have become makes known all things that appear as objects of inquiry for use.
>
> (Bishop, 2011, p. 94)

The final feature of biomedicine identified by Nettleton is the doctrine of specific aetiology, which states that all diseases are caused by identifiable factors (preferably singular ones that can be observed by technical means). This concept has a long history, and though it is widely accepted that most diseases are multifactorial and that, for example, the presence of certain bacteria may be benign in some and pathological in others, this idea still exerts considerable influence in both medical and lay contexts (Deep, 1999). Patients, certainly, often approach disease as a lone intruder operating upon an isolated organ or system within their body, and I think that Lawler (1991, p. 2) is right when she says 'such a viewpoint leaves little space for other aspects of lived experience, such as feelings and emotions, except to the extent that these things can be understood as biologically determined processes'.

Biomedical structures, too, tend to perpetuate the view that biomedical methods are the most deserving of epistemic authority – that all validity surrounding a disease must be drawn from microbiology or histology or physiology or parasitology (or whatever). As Barker (2005, p. 10) writes, 'biomedicine alone is the final arbitrator in determining the existence of a disease. A disease does not exist, so to speak, until the social institution of biomedicine creates a representative diagnostic category.' Not only does this hegemonic approach ignore non-biological factors as discussed above but also acts on the basis that medical knowledge production is 'objective' and without roots in a specific social context, despite much work which has demonstrated otherwise (Fleck, 1981; Latour and Woolgar, 1986).

Where does the *power* of biomedicine come from? – *why* do patients submit to viewing their bodies as machines, and put so much stock by, say, hospital imaging technology? – why do they in many cases arrive at the clinic expecting to be prescribed medication that can treat a part of their body in isolation, confident that such a thing exists? It is because, in part, of the high public esteem in which medicine is held, particularly in relation to defining health and illness and producing knowledge about the body; the structures which determine how doctors think – textbooks, medical schools, hospital practice – are disseminated through personal encounters, media representations, film and fiction, education systems and so on into the general population (Jutel, 2011).

It is also, undoubtably, a result of the huge effectiveness of biomedical approaches to healthcare. Advances in microbiology (and related fields) and their widespread application has indisputably saved a magnitude of lives and vastly increased the power of medicine to react and to heal, and rapid developments in medical technology have allowed us to more accurately detect and observe different stages of previously invisible conditions. In short, a large number of illnesses fit neatly into biomedical understandings of health and sickness, and acute care is more effective than it has been in the history of mankind (Wade and Halligan, 2004). Rising life expectancy, falling infant mortality and steadily increasing clinical outcomes over the second half of the 20th century are due, in large part, to the strengths of the biomedical model in combating disease.

A clear distinction must also be made at this point, as I am keen not to make straw men. Biomedicine is not the same as *medicine*, which can mean many things to many people, be that the divergent strands represented by public health, epidemiology, narrative medicine, doctors, hospitals, or medical science. Likewise, focusing on the medical encounter, it would be caricature to portray doctors as biomedical robots, subjecting patients to their infamous gaze and nothing else. In fact, in might be argued (and has been), that recent trends in biomedical research, delving deep into the genetic makeup of patients, are driving medical science and medical care away from the universals criticised here and towards a much-touted 'personalised medicine' approach that incorporates DNA analysis, wearable medical devices and a far more intimate appreciation of personal microbiomes (Snyder, 2016). Likewise, feminist analysis has revealed the damaging effect that centuries of treating male bodies as the norm has had on the medical care of women, and more attention than ever before is being paid to construct clinical trials which accurately represent the patient groups they will ultimately serve (Dusenbery, 2018).

However, as will become clear, it is often patients who are the real torchbearers of the biomedical viewpoint. And that's what we are discussing here, a viewpoint, a way of seeing the world. One that, while not isomorphic with medicine, nonetheless represents a very real and very significant portion of it, especially among the lay populations I am concerned with in this book, and as such is worthy of independent analysis and criticism.

It is notable that the most strident criticisms of biomedicine have come from sociologists. Their work, as discussed in this chapter, has enabled us to give meaning to health and sickness beyond that which is provided by medical science, and equipped us with tools to challenge the assumptions on which we base our healthcare system. This has provided some support for movements within medicine to establish a broader base for understanding illness, such as the biopsychosocial model, first proposed in the 1970s and often referred to, if apparently little applied (Engel, 1977; Johnson, 2012).

What is lacking however is any concerted effort to respond to biomedicine philosophically. Looking at how the body is understood by practitioners is vital because it determines the way in which health and illness come to be defined within disciplines and as a consequence points towards what is perceived as the best medical response to a situation (Brown and Seddon, 1996). It is also important to recognise how individuals and communities outside of medical practice perceive and experience health and illness as well, and the effect that this has on the sick. I have no doubts that this is as much a philosophical problem as it is a sociological one.

This is because biomedicine is a part of a social process that imparts upon individuals a way of seeing disease, of seeing the body and of seeing bodies. The biomedical body is universal, consistent and constant; its ways of signally distress can be quantified in numerical form; it can be fixed, it can be cured. Corporal regionalism reigns in the clinic. Diseases are malfunctions, external not always (though often) in the necessary sense of having come from outside, but rather in the sense that they are always *external to the norm*. A biomedical body should hold no surprises.

This model seeps into the popular imagination and informs the way that non-medically trained individual encounter illness. To them, disease is visible; ill people *look ill* – they limp, they're pale, their hair falls out, they bleed. Diseases have scientific names because diseases are scientific entities. Disease is always located: you're ill because of this organ or that virus or because of some imbalance in your blood; you are never simply ill. Disease is something to be fought against and triumphed over or it is something to be defeated by; patients get better or they get worse; they do not fluctuate day by day.

This is not to say that this view is malevolent, but rather to state that there are many experiences of sickness which fall outside of these parameters. The patients involved, unsure of their own ideas about their body, conflicted as they are between what they have absorbed and what only they know, cannot find a home for their sensory life in the meanings, explanations and narratives offered by the biomedical model. They are lost, and turn to each other to share the burden of being misunderstood. In the second half of this book, through the words of patients we shall see the reach of the biomedical mindset, extending as it does far beyond the doctor's surgery and into family homes and offices, newspaper articles and online forums, producing sensations of self-doubt and revelatory moments of connection with others, poor communication with doctors and an incomplete understanding of one's self.

This is not the full story, of course, but in part this book will serve as an examination of how resilient the mindset outlined above can be in the face of substantial social changes. The rise of patient organisations, rapid mass communication and normalised self-diagnosis, set against a backdrop of consumer capitalism, the gradual loss of trust in the medical establishment, and a society that valorises personal choice, have produced an environment in which the use of alternative medicine – a strange hodgepodge of new-age holism, cynical exploitation and genuine supplementary care – is widespread and popular, and confidence in traditional sources of authority to deliver results waning.

It might be thought then, that there is sense in which biomedicine is under threat. This is both true and not true. What is fairer to say is that some concrete biomedical structures are being challenged in certain circumstances – that, in other words, there are battlegrounds – but that the way in which they are confronted serves to reinforce rather than diminish the power that the biomedical mindset holds.

We will discuss this later on in more depth, but it will suffice for now to say the following. In the west, it is not unfamiliar to observe the use of biomedical, or scientific-sounding, rhetoric used to sell non-mainstream treatments, and nor is it unusual to witness at alternative drug stalls in America large printed graphs and tables alongside voluminous literature from supposedly reputable journals exalting the values of consuming silver regularly or taking frequent infra-red tent saunas; furthermore, the dissatisfaction most contested illness patients feel with their diagnosis (or lack of one) is its insufficient organicity, not its holism. Or to employ another example, observe the lengths to which patients with depression go to biologise their experiences, preferring to talk of neurochemical imbalances and genetic dispositions than any more general, less physiological relationship between despair, hardship, events, the social environment, the human lot etc., even if the evidence for such a one-dimensional view is limited.

The tension in all of this is not that biomedical authority is under attack, as some may assume, it is that everyone wishes to possess it, regardless of whether they are accepted by the traditional gatekeepers. The 'democratisation' of medicine has not, I believe, effected a shift in our fundamental relationship with the reductionist, mechanist, techno-scientific gaze of modern healthcare, but rather given us more tools to, when it benefits us socially and psychologically, siphon off parts of it and call it our own.

In the next chapter I will look at how philosophers have responded to some of the questions raised above, or not responded, as the case may be.

Chapter 3

Definitions of disease

Introduction

In 1992, Arthur Caplan published a famous paper in *Theoretical Medicine and Bioethics* entitled 'Does the philosophy of medicine exist?' (Caplan, 1992). Within it he detailed various necessary features of a 'field' and concluded, broadly to his own disappointment, that philosophy of medicine did not satisfy those conditions. Therefore, it should not yet be considered a discipline in its own right and did not as such 'exist'. His demarcation criteria were that a field must be integrated into cognate areas of study; it should have a distinct and wrangled-over canon of literature; and that there ought to be present some key puzzles or vital questions which form the centrepieces of the main debates. Philosophy of medicine, in his view, failed to make the grade in any of these three categories.[1]

It is the first and last of Caplan's criteria with which I am most interested here. He argued that philosophy of medicine is too removed from practice, and that philosophers do not do enough to place themselves as loud, useful voices in relation to medicine. It is this baton I would like to raise here. I broadly agree with his suggestion that philosophy of medicine is too insular and inward-looking, and that its proponents have not done enough to make themselves relevant.

Then there is the question of central problems. Caplan (1992, p. 73) conceded that the debate surrounding 'health' and 'disease' comes closest to passing his test, but argues that these do not constitute enough to 'transform a mixed set of ruminations into an actual field'. In the years since his paper these concepts have been developed to a greater extent, perhaps even to the level of complexity which might represent bona fide field-hood, but that is not what I am concerned with. What I would like to focus on mainly in this

1 His overall thrust is fairly irrelevant to this work, and my position is closest to Stempsey's (2008) retrospective and roughly inclusive view. As such, the strength or weakness of Caplan's position is not under discussion here, and I do not wish my use of his paper to be taken as a tacit endorsement of his views. I am using his work here as a springboard for discussion, not as an item for analysis itself.

chapter is philosophical attempts to define disease, the underlying motivations for such efforts and the extent to which these could be considered a success. A subsidiary aim is to demonstrate the poor conceptual tools we are left with from such efforts when it comes to approaching contested illness.

Disease is a central problem

I agree with Caplan, insofar as the definition of disease is a problem which is and has been central to the philosophy of medicine (as do others: Nordenfelt, 2013; Lemoine, 2013). Partly, its importance appears to be derived from the benefits that clear demarcation criteria might bring. For a start, distinguishing between health and disease appears a necessary prerequisite for the just distribution of limited resources within any healthcare infrastructure. The allocation of benefits, material, medical or social, seems to rely on someone or something being able to tell disease from non-disease. There are as well a large range of controversial cases which come to mind, such as those that fall on the fine line between treatment and enhancement – whether we should then treat body dysmorphic disorder with cosmetic surgery for example – or indeed the demarcation between treatment and non-necessary amputation, which is often sought by those with body identity integrity disorder, and both of these troublesome distinctions could, in theory, benefit from greater clarity surrounding 'disease' and its hypothetical opposite 'non-disease'.[2] The special interest here of course, contested illnesses, would seem to gain greatly from proper categorisation, as the uncertainty that exists at present bleeds credibility from patient's experience.[3] In any case, the examples touched upon above are just a few of the topics which could be plausibly profit from a thorough and sophisticated elucidation of the term 'disease'.

So yes, it would appear that answering, or attempting to answer, the question 'what is disease?' serves a useful purpose. However, in this chapter I will argue the opposite. Attempting to define disease in a universal, closed sense, is a futile exercise. What's more, it is one which gestates further futile exercises, in the form of a prolonged theoretical tussle from which no winner is ever likely to emerge. My argument is that philosophers who attempt a universal definition of disease, one which is able to sharply demarcate disease, are caught in an impossible bind. Maël Lemoine blames the procedural restraints of conceptual analysis for this, and I will explore his position. But I will also posit that there are other factors that make their attempts unlikely to be fruitful.

2 I make a distinction here between 'disease' and 'non-disease' not only because defining 'health', which most would take instinctively to be the opposite, has its own troubled definition history, but also because all that is not disease *is* 'non-disease', whereas plenty which is not disease is also not health.

3 Though it remains to be seen what exactly would happen should their situations be judged or assigned to not be 'disease'.

I will show that given their aims, philosophers of disease either intend their theories to be descriptive or normative. In the case of the former, it is highly improbable, given the desire to generate a set of stipulations which includes all which is disease and excludes all which is not, that they will be successful. This is due to the sheer diversity of entities that might be considered 'disease' and some pressing but unconsidered epistemic issues. The creation of such a schema rests upon a necessary essentialism about disease which does not come close to enjoying adequate empirical support. I call this the vast magnitude argument, and I believe it applies even if you try and restrict disease entities to something that appears fairly common-sense and self-contained (say, 'medical' usage) as well as to broader normativist theories of disease. For the latter, the normative angle, it is simply that their conceptualisations carry little weight and make no strong claims as to why we should respect their authority. I call this the justification gap argument. This argument has two strands: a theoretical deficiency which I will contrast with bio-ethics and a practical element, which is that the words spoken in philosophy of medicine fail to echo anywhere else.

Furthermore, I will argue that following this approach has a nefarious influence on the discipline as a whole. Most notably, the focus on all-encompassing theories of disease steers problem selection away from practice and into the arms of pedantry. To quote Caplan (1992, p. 72) again, recent work on disease definition has done little to challenge the idea that 'the philosophy of medicine looks from afar like an intellectual island' with no 'connections to other parts of the intellectual map'. Using Illari and Russo's (2014) taxonomy of counterexamples, I will discuss how this problem might be approached and how plausible new directions in philosophy of disease would seem.

Before I do this, though, it would be worth outlining the field, questioning the key assumptions and aims of the philosophers, detailing some of the more influential positions that have been taken, and focusing on a few of the ways that people have approached the big questions surrounding disease: what is it and how should it be defined? I will make this section brief as there already exists voluminous literature on the topic and what is more pertinent here is how we move past the current strictures of debate.

Why define disease?

What is the purpose of achieving a succinct and self-contained definition of disease? As with any 'defining of terms' discourse, the possible reasons are varied. Practical concerns, for example. Surely there is a straightforward, almost bureaucratic benefit to defining disease? After all, with the large amounts of public and private money spent on healthcare, there must be an incentive to strengthen our ability to adequately draw a line between who or what deserves resources. A strong, formulaic definition that could be referred to or imbued in practice would seem to serve a useful role. Certainly there are no shortage of controversial cases that would apparently benefit from some appeal to a higher adjudicator, especially in state-funded and distributed healthcare.

Armed with such a definition, perhaps we could make progress on, for example, deciding whether people who eat fatty foods and exercise little become *sufferers* of obesity and therefore deserve access to relatively expensive surgical procedures.[4] Indeed, politically, a strong and reductive disease definition could be wielded against medicalisation, over-diagnosis and fears of boundary creep.

Along with distributing finite resources, a complete definition of disease would allow us to resolve some of the more fluid issues surrounding distribution, such as the allocation of sick roles, sympathy and the validation of an individual's embodied experience. These contentious and often painful battles to grab and hold on to legitimacy again could profit from reference to a higher, codified arbiter. Something like a gold standard in demarcation might play this role and be held up by those on the blurry edge of disease like a certificate, a qualification that entitles them to be sick.

Diagnostically, it could be argued that a single, useable definition of disease would enable healthcare professionals to make better decisions in the clinic, protecting their decision-making process from the sometimes nefarious influence of pharmaceutical companies, patient groups and insurance companies.

It may be the case that a slight codification of demarcation criteria could be achieved while retaining some of the plurality of the current, organic, case-by-case, institution-by-institution system. That is to say, we could move towards having a regular set of demarcation criteria to be used economically in terms of resource allocation, while generating a different set for clinical situations and so on, which would still reduce greatly the number of stipulations for disease status in use.

Finally, to return to the aims of philosophers, there is a conceptual mapping aspect to all of this. Put simply, disease exists in variant forms throughout institutions, cultures, individuals and time. It is real in the sense that people believe in its reality. Indeed, despite the high variance with which it is found over a great multitude of different contexts, its core 'reality' is for the most part undiminished. And so there is a solid and understandable drive to describe and explain this phenomenon conceptually, and integrate it into a nexus of related concepts, as is the case in other parts of philosophy for other entities. Whether this pursuit is a directly fruitful endeavour is not always the point; sometimes it is enough that the ideas were wrestled with and that the picture became slightly more in focus. Often the true yield of such work is initially obscure, and sometimes conceptual debates have surprising and pleasant outcomes far from the theoretical realm.

I am not, however, at all convinced by the above arguments. I believe they rely on things that will not come to pass, and an oversimplified misreading of

4 For an extended and fascination discussion of these sorts of questions, see Elliott (2004).

clinical practice, and that, for philosophy, they have unintended and deleterious consequences. My objections will be clarified, but I have included these potential motivations for attempting the task here so that we can better analyse the success of various responses on their own terms.

Is this, then, what philosophers are trying to achieve? Are they hoping to define disease in order to solve or advance some of the problems that I have outlined above?

Maël Lemoine (2013) looked in detail at three important writers on this topic – Christopher Boorse, Lennart Nordenfelt and Jerome Wakefield – and discussed the motivations that drive philosophers of medicine to attack this problem. Though he found that each had a closely related but distinct 'major goal', which tended toward the broad and vague, he concluded that alongside this came concerns similar to those I have raised. These relate directly to the sort of advantageous consequences they perceive their definitions to have, for example eliminating false positives in diagnosis and resolving disputed or borderline cases. They also retain a strong link to the things generally considered to be 'disease', at least insofar as they represent a considerably large set of cases that must be satisfactorily assimilated for a definition to be considered successful. Finally, it would appear to be the case that some level of conceptual coherence is a worthwhile goal in its own right for these thinkers, and that work which is able to reconcile the different notions of 'disease', 'health', 'mental illness', 'injury', etc. which are currently present in the literature is deserving of attention.

It seems evident, therefore, that philosophers see themselves as having clear motivations for doing this kind of work, and that they anticipate benefits emerging from their attempts. Before I go into detail as to why I take a contrary view, it will be useful to describe the main positions that individuals take in this field.

Outline of the field

Within the definition of disease debate (and discussion of health more widely), there have over the last thirty years emerged two loose groupings of theorists, shoe-horned into what philosophers love to call a 'false dichotomy' (Carel and Cooper, 2013).[5] It is known as such due largely to the coherence and consistency of one thinker, Christopher Boorse, in the light of whom disparate opponents begin to seem united.

5 Though many have commented on the convoluted nature of this divide: for example see Kingma (2014); in this section I have deliberately attempted to narrow the literature analysed to those working on the 'disease definition problem'. I did this because it is probably the largest glut of literature in the field around a single topic and therefore worthy of attention and because incorporating the work done at its edges would involve significant detours which, enlightening as they may be, I do not have space for here.

His ideas have formed the basis of the naturalist tradition, which positions disease as a series of entities which can be uncovered in a 'value-free' manner (Kingma, 2017). In essence, naturalists argue that disease (along with health) is a concept which exists in the real world (that is to say, it *really exists*, irrespective of our theorising about it) and can be described without necessitating the involvement of evaluative elements. Specifically, the usual arguments employed are that disease is revealed in a body by a statistical abnormality, measured scientifically, which indicates that natural function (usually framed in evolutionary terms) has been impaired. Bodies consist of systems which have specific life-maintaining goals, and a departure from the normal functioning of these systems (which is not harmless or beneficial) amounts to a disease state. Conscious of some of the basic problems of normality, these statistical deviations are only considered significant if they are anomalous for the type (age, sex, ethnicity, etc.) of person that experiences them. So, a young, ethnically Chinese woman who is lactose intolerant and flushes red while drinking has little wrong with her (presuming that a biological aversion to dairy and struggling to metabolising alcohol are the only thing 'abnormal' about her body). These categories or sub-groups are generally referred to as reference classes.

These disease classifications are regarded as 'value-free' because they supposedly require no subjective decision making. They are argued to exist independently of normative judgement: they simply tell us whether something is a disease, not whether it is good or bad to have it. Most naturalists expand this to a two-stage process, whereby we first identify biological malfunctions (facts) and then indulge in normative discussions about what this means (whether the person is suffering, whether we should medically intervene, etc.) This approach is still a naturalist position because conceptual priority is given to the objective, organic descriptions and because those descriptions are assumed to be real and value free in a concrete and meaningful way.

Across from these naturalists sit the normativists. They take a different tack regarding the objectivity of biological facts; in the case of disease they believe classifications to be 'value-laden'. These philosophers are placed together because their ideas promote a fundamentally subjective element to disease definition, insofar as they believe calling something a disease necessarily involves making a normative judgement. That is, when deciding whether or not something is a disease, we are forced to make a statement about phenomena which does not and cannot speak for itself. To call upon the words of Temkin (1977), who, as so often, said it best, disease can only exist within 'man's moral universe, when its occurrence within a scheme of creation and right and wrong are accounted for'. However, beyond these fairly vague appeals to the subjectivity and judgement involved in defining disease, it is problematic to place all normativists in the same category as the positions they promote can be quite divergent. There is enough variety and disagreement on this side of the discussion that it is questionable whether maintaining normativism as a distinct position is still worthwhile. Normativism means many things to many people.

It is important at this point to highlight that the general, fundamental level at which most of the disputes between naturalists and normativists take place is a conceptual one. This field is largely concerned with the theoretical nature of disease, and not with how disease is applied in a social or lay context, nor even necessarily by medical practitioners (although, confusingly, this is often presented as evidence for the desirability of choosing one theory over another). So, for naturalists, the core features of a disease relate to function and dysfunction as understood as statistical deviation, and for normativists these vital components are defined by some form of evaluative process.

A few interesting and dissenting voices have been raised which question, as I do, the value in pursuing this problem *at all*, or at least in the way that it has been done thus far. Lemoine has highlighted the ways in which this debate is positioned as one of straightforward conceptual analysis, which in turn dictates the sort of theories, evidence and arguments that are permissible and constrains the possible outcomes.[6] His examination of the 'rules of the game' are a welcome excavation and I shall examine his thoughts. Hesslow (1993) famously took a stronger position, arguing that the weight given to possessing a disease concept is illusionary and distracting, and that the importance of such a definition to clinical practice is vastly overstated. I will revisit his arguments later on in this chapter.

Elsewhere, Kidd, Carel and others have tried to break with this tradition by proposing and debating the utility of developing a modern phenomenology of illness (e.g. Kidd, 2012; Kidd, 2013; Carel, 2014). I will examine the phenomenological position at greater length below, but it is important to note here that these thinkers argue from the same sense of frustration that I do. Of the conceptual inadequacy of both the medical and philosophical worlds, Carel writes:

> Because of my training as a philosopher, my experiences pushed me to reflect abstractly on health and illness: what these concepts mean and how best to understand them. But when I started my research I found that the language and concepts routinely used to describe illness are inappropriate, incomplete and often misleading. I became increasingly aware of the impoverished language used in the medical world I encountered, which, in turn, led me to suspect that an impoverished concept of illness was in the background.
>
> (Carel, 2008, pp. 8–9)

I will now provide a brief description of a variety of different positions within this field, in order to give a sense of the sorts of arguments that are employed and the types of responses that could be considered representative.

6 Schwartz (2014) also makes this point.

Different ways of defining disease – the naturalism of Christopher Boorse

It is customary in this debate to start any discussion on disease definition by outlining and then criticising some aspect of Boorse's naturalist position, as his is the longest standing and most disputed theory of disease. In fact, I would go as far as to say that critical interactions between definitions of disease where one theorist does not position themselves in contrast to Boorse are rare (one exception being Schramme, 2007). So central is he that Thomas Schramme (ibid., p. 565) adapts Nozick's comment about Rawls to say 'it can be demanded that philosophers of medicine must now either work within Boorse's theory or explain why not'.

As discussed above, Boorse's naturalism is centred around dysfunction and uncovering biological facts about disease. The bio-statistical theory (the BST), as his ideas are commonly called, rests on three main concepts. The first is physiological function, which is defined as the causal contribution a system (nervous, respiratory, circulatory, etc.) makes towards biological goals (survival and reproduction for example). The second is the idea of a reference class, described above. These reference classes define what is considered typical for the individual under investigation. The third is a statistical concept, the idea of organic statistical abnormality, which helps to delimit pathological from normal activity.

Arranged in tandem with each other, these three ideas give us a fairly clear, if not specific, notion of Boorse's theory. A disease is therefore present if there is a statistical abnormality, the result of which impairs some aspect of a person's physiological functioning and is untypical for that individual's reference class. Or, as he (Boorse, 1997, p. 8) puts it: 'a disease is a type of internal state which is … an impairment of normal functional ability, i.e., a reduction of one or more functional abilities below typical efficiency'.

These fundamental ideas and the places that they lead have been attacked for the best part of half a century. Almost every aspect of his theory has been critiqued, the most effective arguments being those which focus on the improbability of uncovering his basic criteria in a value-free manner (Smart, 2016). Reference classes are not strong enough to be natural kinds and neither is physiological functioning, even dressed in evolutionary clothing, objectively easy to determine. Classic statistical issues of normality and line-drawing problems also stalk Boorse. Of further difficulty to him are several examples of diseases that seem straightforward under his classification but are not considered to be diseases in general medical contexts. Homosexuality is a case in point here, as it would appear to be unequivocally a disease state under his schema, a state of affairs very much out of step with contemporary thinking. These criticisms hold especial weight considering that Boorse purports the symmetry of his theory with medical usage to be one of its great advantages.

These complaints are strong, and it is not clear that Boorse has been able to adequately account for some or any of them, though he has responded to critics periodically (Boorse, 1997; Boorse, 2014). All that sometimes seems to hold his ideas afloat is the intuition that disease *is* related intrinsically to human biology. His is, after all, the theory which ties itself most firmly to the organic and the natural. Beyond this indefatigable connection, however, which the majority of thinkers likewise wish to retain, all or almost all of his arguments are contentious and have been convincingly challenged.

Nevertheless, despite these criticisms, he is still at the forefront of the field. *Why* he remains so important, so vital, so referenced, is difficult to tell. This is particularly interesting given the imbalance of support and criticism in the literature. His ideas have been rebuked and dismissed on many occasions, in a manner that in many other areas of philosophy or general academic discourse would seem adequate. George Khushf has also noted this apparent enigma, writing:

> The scholarly response to Boorse has been vigorous and, at the same time, puzzling. Few accept his disease concept. When Boorse published a rebuttal to his many critics [in 1997], his bibliography lists well over a hundred such critics, and a literature search on the current philosophical debate indicates his work is among the most cited. Despite the broad consensus against his view, nearly everyone feels the need to return to Boorse and criticize him again. Why? This is the puzzling part.
>
> (Khushf, 2007, p. 19)

I can offer two explanations for this.

The first is that Boorse represents a convenient foil. His work is continually discredited because it is easy to criticise from a constructivist or loosely constructivist position which questions his basic assumptions surrounding normality and reference class objectivity and it is always nice to begin a paper with a refutation that strengthens your own position.

My second speculation is that Boorse is relevant not because of the philosophical rigour of his theories, but because these theories are the closest thing we have to a medical viewpoint. Therefore the importance of his thoughts is derived from their isomorphic or near-isomorphic relationship with practice. He himself has claimed this to be true, and it certainly should make us pause and consider the value of the BST in a different way. If this is indeed nearer to how medical practitioners view disease, then what can we do with this knowledge? What effect might that mindset have on patients, on procedure, on insurance? Medical epistemologists know well the shortfalls of applying general theories to individuals, and it is fair to say that debates like this (i.e. what do practitioners consider disease, how do they arrive at this, etc.) are common across lots of different arenas of medical decision making and knowledge production (Solomon, 2015). This, if anything, adds value and relevance to the BST: if it is not only a way of conceptualising disease but a way that disease is actually conceptualised in practice, then all sorts of interesting work can proceed.[7] Unfortunately, not much has been done on the BST outside of philosophy. As it is, the work remains strangely important and an obligatory introductory sentence for pretty much everyone working on the philosophy of disease who isn't Christopher Boorse.

Normativism

Normativism does not have such a figurehead, but rather a multitude of theorists orbiting its own central postulate: disease is about value judgements. A proper analysis of health and disease suggests, to them, that what we label with these terms tells us more about our own norms than it does about some biological reality. Thus, desirable states become something to which to aspire, and which we associate with health, and likewise undesirable circumstances become called diseases.

There are many general criticisms which are offered to this simplistic representation of normativism. It immediately appears too inclusive, and, rather than resolving controversies, seems to actively encourage them (alcoholism, obesity, ageing, etc. all become straightforward seeming disease states). Furthermore, it renders disease a relativistic beast, entirely at the whim of the society it is found in, and subsequently allows for historical (and contemporary) instances of persecution-by-medicine to be unproblematically justified. Stock examples from this criticism include homosexuals, political dissidents in the Soviet Union and slaves who ran away from plantations, all of whom were at one point considered diseased because of overt ideological biases present in the surrounding medical communities and societies at large. Finally, normativism of the strongest sort breaks the intuitive bond with nature, the idea that there is some intangible or rather unquantifiable but supremely real connection between disease states and biology.

The above sketch is superficial, so to get a better idea of the sorts of arguments normativists put forward, let us look at Rachel Cooper's ideas. She sets out her aims in a way that is fairly typical of normativist accounts:

> I suggest that a neat account of disease cannot be achieved. By 'disease' we aim to pick out a variety of conditions that through being painful, disfiguring or disabling are of interest to us as people. No biological account of disease can be provided because this class of conditions is by

7 It may be the case, in fact, that many of those who criticise Boorse do so *because* of the similarities between his view and that of the dominant biomedical model, and in criticising his position they are raising broader issues with the way that medical science classifies disease. This is not made explicit anywhere that I can see, but I nonetheless think it might be an interesting avenue of inquiry.

> its nature anthropocentric and corresponds to no natural class of conditions in the world.
>
> I shall argue that by disease we mean a condition that it is a bad thing to have, that is such that we consider the afflicted person to have been unlucky, and that can potentially be medically treated. All three criteria must be fulfilled for a condition to be a disease.
>
> (Cooper, 2002, p. 271)

From here she goes on to explain each category in detail, describing how she sees her account to be more a synthesis of previous normativist writing than a novel theory of disease.[8] A person is sick if they have something which is considered bad to have, which allows her to negate some of the criticisms thrown at naturalists, such as the classification of homosexuality in contemporary society. Her second postulate, that a diseased person must be considered unlucky, is basically a normative version of a reference class. As she says of her definition of an unlucky individual, she is talking about someone 'that is, roughly, worse off than the majority of humans of the same sex and age'. This allows her to skirt around the normality question and account for people with disabilities. Her final criterion is that the condition must be *potentially* medically treated. That is to say, either now or hypothetically at some point in the future, we might be able to medically intervene in order to alleviate the disease. This acts as a blade which cuts disease away from economic and social problems a person might have which would fulfil her first two categories.

Overall, her account is much more nebulous than any naturalist view would allow, and this is a problem faced by many normativist attempts. Under her 'bad to have' category she admits the subjective and individual nature of this description may lead to some cases where a seemingly diseased person does not think themselves to 'have something bad' (such as in examples of schizophrenia where individuals have vivid and enjoyable hallucinations that form a part of their identity). She tries to pull herself out of this quandary by arguing that in the great majority of cases there will be no disagreement (a statement itself open to question), but it remains a firm counterargument.

On her second point, even she admits that 'being unlucky' is 'medically unsophisticated', and I think the conceptual messiness of this argument detracts from the overall credibility of her view. Her final criterion, about potential medical treatment, seems rather indeterminate, and it's not clear that a theory with so many overly variable components could be considered a strong conceptual challenger to a naturalist account. It is also the case, as Cooper recognises, that her schema tends towards inclusiveness, to the point where things such as unwanted pregnancy are cast as diseases. If this account is demonstrative of anything, it is that it remains easier to criticise Boorse than to suggest a viable alternative.

8 Which is precisely why I feel it is a good example to discuss.

I hope that the above discussion has given a flavour of the sort of arguments put forward by naturalists and normativists, as well as a few of the stock critiques of such views. Clearly, I feel that both schools of thought are unsuccessful in their attempts. This is not, however, through lack of trying or theoretical sophistication, but rather because from the beginning they have set themselves a question which is impossible to answer. It is to this conceptual bind that we now turn.

The reasons why definitions of disease fail

One commonality of most attempts to define disease is their all-encompassing nature. The very act of delimitation in this instance is necessarily one that requires completeness; the purpose of creating such a definition in the first place is to arrange phenomena neatly, or as neatly as possible, into a box labelled 'disease' and to make sure nothing else gets put in by mistake. Above and beyond other motivations, this aim is, I believe, central to the conceptual exercise that is being engaged with here. Quite simply, there would be little point in producing a list of stipulations that was only able to demarcate certain phenomena as disease but not others. The two key assumptions made by anyone using this approach is that disease *can* be captured by a single definition and, by extension, that all diseases have some fundamental similarity.

It is true that some philosophers try to be more 'universal' than others: Boorse restricts himself to what he regards as medical uses of the term whereas someone like Nordenfelt (2013) tries to explain not just human conditions but also animal and plant diseases with his ideas. Even at their most restricted, however, the theories of disease that are found in the literature are still extensive and dynamic. They are intended as a set of postulates which can be tested against our current pool of examples but which will also prove to be accurate into the future as new cases are assimilated. In theory, there is no limit at all to the number of entities they could be expected to describe. There is, then, more than a hint of universalism about them.

Once formulated, these definitions *have* to be either descriptive or normative.[9] That is, they have to either be an attempt to describe what disease means within socially existing parameters – be it medical uses of the term, intuitive interpretations of 'undeniable' disease or some other broad categorisation – or they are a suggestion of ways in which we might define disease for whatever purpose. On the whole, it would seem that most of the theories thrown around in this debate are trying to be descriptive. They are attempts to articulate succinctly a pre-existing category of things, a grouping commonly recognised and frequently encountered but currently ill-defined.

9 Lemoine draws this distinction as one between 'description' and 'stipulation', but our uses are similar.

However, the purely descriptive approach described here clashes with some of the aims described above (resource allocation, diagnostic clarity, etc.), which suggests that there must be a normative element involved if any theory is to fulfil these objectives. In any case, both of these possibilities (descriptive and normative) are, I believe, doomed to fail. I will deal with these two options in turn and examine why they might not be successful.

Descriptive failure

It is clear that the majority of disease definition literature purports to be at least partially descriptive. Certainly, many theorists draw extensively on examples of disease to support their ideas and use the same reservoir to attack their opponents. A counterexample that does not accord with a theory, drawn from either the real-world or a similar but hypothetical world, is the most common form of criticism offered. At the very least, the best indicator that we seem to have of the strength of a theory of disease in this context is the extent to which it accurately overlays some external map of disease which pre-exists in the world.

In response to this I put it that there are simply too many *things* that count as disease for this to ever be a successful project. Even within a strictly confined theoretical space, the vast magnitude of different types of entities that could make a claim to disease status is staggering. It is not so much that there are so many diseases as it is that there are so many ways of thinking about disease and so many ways that disease is thought about. If we were to try and, as some do, strip away from the fatty edges of disease all common usage of the term and cut from the centre some form of solid terminology only used by medical professionals, I still believe we would be left with this problem. Different areas of medicine deal with disease definition in a variety of ways. Disease can exist on a spectrum between normal and pathological or as the presence of a particular bacterium or because of the discovery of certain cells. It may be purely symptomatic. It can be acute or chronic, universal or extremely rare. Sometimes what may be disease in one individual is not a disease in another. Sometimes what may be disease in one culture is not a disease somewhere else. Most diseases appear to be harmful, but not all are. Having a disease may prevent another disease. Some diseases are fully subsumed into a biomedical causal matrix, but many can and are not. This indeterminacy goes on. What is important here is that both the conventional, common-language usage of the term and more specialist application produce a hopelessly manifold array of entities. Indeed, this is precisely the reason why counterexamples are so often employed in the disease definition debate: because there is an incredibly diverse set from which to draw from, and there is simply no way of accounting for all of them without falling into the trap of including that which appears clearly to not be disease. We can define diseases, and do so regularly, using a number of different methods depending on the purpose of our criteria, but we cannot define disease.[10]

To my mind there is no better evidence for this position than the inability of philosophers to make progress on this problem over a fairly long amount of time. As Kingma (2013, p. 37) states, 'thirty years of literature has failed to deliver an answer' to the disease question. I would state this in even firmer terms: the debate has digressed in a few different directions but the fundamental issues remain the same, remain fundamentally unresolved and there is scarce evidence to suggest that this will change through the continued use of current methods. It may be that the reason so little ground has been made is because the target itself keeps moving, as 'the concepts of health and disease have become problematic in ways that are unprecedented' (Carel and Cooper, 2013, p. 2).

This is owing to, among other things, the rise of economic and social protection for those with diseases, the challenging of normality and perceptions of pathological states by disability campaigners, the growth in size and influence of patient groups, the discussion around enhancement, sex change operations and the increasing medicalisation of previously non-medical conditions. But even if this is the case, a rapidly changing medico-social environment underlines further the futility of attempting a statement of complete conceptual containment, especially as philosophers are not on the whole trying to provide a snapshot but rather something more dynamic. If historical and hypothetical examples are to be employed as counterexamples, then it is reasonable to expect that a condition of a theory is that it not only apply to the present but also to the past and the future.

Schwartz has made a similar point to those described above, contrasting scientific reality with the essentialist aspirations of philosophers:

> As scientists have acquired better and better understanding of diseases and their causes, they find not a unifying microstructure, as for gold or water, but variation. While many have sought an essence that all and only diseases share, this quest has been blocked at every step by variability and heterogeneity. Any definition that would draw a sharp line through all conditions, determining for each whether it is a disease or not, looks like the imposition of a decision, rather than the application of a discovery.
>
> (Schwartz, 2007, p. 59)

What Schwartz is suggesting here is that the philosophy of disease has proceeded on the basis that diseases are natural kinds of some form or other.

10 The retort to this might be that the ICD-10 appears to do a good job of defining disease. I would say that this is indeed true, but it is constructed on a case-by-case basis rather than an essentialist one. There are no necessary criteria for being included but there is a staggering amount of diversity.

While this is an angle that has been used to attack naturalist conceptions of disease, most notably by Reznek (1987), I would like to employ it here to criticise the heart of descriptive theories of disease: their reliance on a regularity and uniqueness to diseases that does not seem empirically sound. This regularity is admittedly twofold. Naturalists appear to presume a physical, biostatistical reality to disease which is easy to criticise as a natural kind argument, and has been so, as I have described above. Normativists do not believe in this form of measurable unity, and indeed it is this which in many ways separates them most from naturalists. They do however, also lean upon a different sort of universalism: that there is enough consistency in our agreed set of disease examples (and indeed that enough of us agree on said examples) that it is possible to design a framework capable of capturing them without capturing anything else.

Now, this consistency might have little to do with microbiology, pathophysiology, evolutionary function, variations from a norm, etc., but it nonetheless requires the presence of some underlying and particular quality or qualities, which are found in diseases as mediated by us and not in non-diseases. Thus is it that in the standard normativist approaches, their routine stipulations (causes harm, unlucky for the individual, etc.) *become* the universal features of disease. It is just that these concrete features are framed as instrumental rather than statistical or structural, and the level of discovery is moved from the actual world, or 'the facts', to the tools we use to uncover them. Both naturalist and normativist theories of disease are then to some degree universalist schemas, and struggle on that basis to account for the distinctly non-universal features of disease.

Normative failure

So, what if we change the intention, then, and say that these theories are not meant to be descriptive, but rather normative? They might still reasonably gain some credibility from descriptive accuracy, but largely their success would be found in their ability to achieve some predetermined goals, such as reducing diagnostic creep or resolving controversial cases. An example of this is the work of Thomas Schramme, who argues that naturalism can provide us with a fairly stable and useful concept of disease which is a necessary guard against medicalisation. In fact, Boorse's original intention was to kick back against what he called the 'psychiatric turn' under whose influence medicine was, in his view, dangerously encroaching on the territory until then occupied by social morality. Another advantage of reformulating disease definitions as normative exercises is that they are freed from the vast magnitude argument discussed above: if you are stating what *should* be rather than what *is*, then you are apparently no longer tied down by the tyranny of examples. However, you still have to provide a justification for your theory – as to why it is a good way of classifying phenomena, what we gain by organising things in this way and how exactly this would work in practice. It is here that this normative framing fails to convince.

It is rare to see explicit justification given to the usefulness of choosing one model or theory of disease over another. The benefits of possessing a clear concept of disease in general are often highlighted, but very little space is afforded to justifying the adoption of one particular view in light of its non-descriptive advantages. The one salient factor that splits theories is their relative ability to accurately reflect intuitive feelings about what disease is and what a disease looks like, *not* any values relating to applicability or outcomes. So, in fact, defining disease is often more like a clever parlour game than a debate with implications for real life. When Caplan spoke about the philosophy of medicine being removed from practice, this is what he had in mind.

Yet there are times when philosophers have stated, or at least hinted at, normative aims. While Boorse maintains for the most part that his account is a descriptive one, and uses the Standard Nomenclature of Diseases and Operations as a guide by which to judge his success, he also stipulates that some universal conditions such as periodontal disease should not be considered disease states, which belies a normative aspect to his work. Cooper (2002, p. 278) too highlights a notable discrepancy between her theory and existing convention by arguing that 'we still think of unwanted pregnancy as not being a disorder because our intuitions lag behind changes in the disorder-status of a condition', suggesting that there is at least some element of her thinking which is out of step with common assumptions but simultaneously not a problem for her theory.

What is more important than this however, is that even if philosophers of medicine *were* solely concerned with the practical application of their ideas, and presented theories as explicitly designed to capture disease in a socially useful way, it is highly doubtful that they would be very successful in challenging and changing medical practice. Medicine, for all intents and purposes, defines disease. Individuals are tested and diagnosed and treated in their hordes daily. A long-standing, sophisticated and, though fragmented, effective infrastructure exists across the world to do precisely that. There is nothing to suggest that a universal theory of disease would have any great effect on clinical medicine.

A hypothetical example might make this point clearer. Say, for whatever reason, a 'new' disease emerged. Social infrastructure begins to coalesce around it: patient advocacy groups are formed, conferences are held, medical responses are researched. In countries with largely private healthcare systems, insurance companies sit up and take notice – is this something they should be covering? Now, this condition is controversial and potentially expensive. People who believe they suffer from it clash with individuals who deny them. Who would we look to in order to solve this controversy and to resolve the conflict? Which bodies carry epistemic and ontological authority in these situations? Certainly not, under current conditions, philosophers. It is difficult to conceive of a situation where a new illness would be cross-referenced with some list of philosophical stipulations in order to decide whether or not it was adequately disease-like.

This is not to say that philosophy cannot speak to and help us understand medicine, or that it cannot gently nudge and cajole the dominant modes of thinking. It is just that in this specific circumstance – formulating a self-contained theory of disease – any claim to practical consequences is probably overstated. Diseases, on the whole, are already defined adequately, and those that aren't are unlikely to be helped by a universal theory of disease. This is because an essentialist proposition that emerges from a theoretical, philosophical base has no credibility in competition with definitions that grow out of biomedical structures. It will not carry more weight in controversial cases than medical opinion or patient views.

A contrast can be drawn here between the philosophy of medicine and bioethics (which is a distinction that Caplan also makes). The history of bioethics in the second half of the 20th century and the fledgling decades of this one serves to remind us how influential and important reflective, philosophical thought can be. Bioethics, in all its complicated permutations, reframes classic ethical questions and brings arguments to bear on cases as they develop. Sitting as it does at the intersection between medical practice, theory and law, this is a discipline fully integrated to other cognate areas of study and administration.

In the International Bioethics Committee, it possess a forum whose authority is recognised worldwide and all of the UNESCO member states have adopted the Universal Declaration on Bioethics and Human Rights, which was unveiled against a backdrop of a 'great number of existing international guidelines, statements and declarations relating to bioethics' (Andorno, 2007, p. 150). Since membership of UNESCO stretches to 195 countries, this is a sizeable achievement in terms of global influence. There are also many declarations which deal with more specific areas of the discipline, such as the UN Declaration on Human Cloning or the UNESCO Universal Declaration on the Human Genome and Human Rights.

The movement has been criticised (though what movement is without critics), but these criticisms are levelled at its intrusiveness into scientific autonomy, the correct level at which to administrate conventions, whether a certain body or other possesses a mandate to grant it authority, the effectiveness of non-binding declarations, etc., and not aimed at its core relevance. The fact remains that bioethics sits in sharp contrast with the philosophy of medicine as an academic subject that has an impact on behaviour and alters policy while remaining in large part a theoretical, normative discipline driven by a long history of deep thinking.

The road to influence and to relevance may well be harder for philosophers of medicine. It is not immediately obvious in which ways they can and should assert themselves, as recent historical precedence is lacking. Some things are clear though. The temptation to remain insular in our work, to offer critique without broader vision, is one which must be consciously avoided and different questions must be asked in order to return to the realm of relevance.

Other critics

In this section I have argued that any universal theory of disease is necessarily either descriptive or normative, and that both approaches, whether actual or hypothetical, fail. This is because there exists too much diversity in what people consider to be disease entities and because there is no suitable justification given that would likely influence medicine to accept and adapt to normative suggestions made by philosophy. You either say what *is* and you're wrong or you say what *ought to be* and nobody listens to you. However, I am not the first to critique this field, and other theorists' views strengthen my argument.

A long-standing criticism that covers some of the same ground as I have comes from Germund Hesslow, who in 1993 asked the question 'do we need a concept of disease?' (Hesslow, 1993). His central argument is that the importance of possessing a clear disease concept is illusionary and that philosophy's obsession with this 'conceptual straightjacket' obscures the fact that it makes very little difference to clinical decision-making. What he contends is that since we treat things that aren't diseases and don't treat things that are, as well as provide medical provision to some degree based on economic grounds, then the best way of formulating medical decision-making is as a cost–benefit analysis, rather than anything crucially reliant on an abstract and universal view of disease. His central point is well made: having a clear definition of disease as a whole is not essential to medical care, where other factors take precedence.

Some thinkers have suggested problems within this field are largely caused by the constraints of the conceptual analysis used to try and answer the original question. As Leen De Vreese (2016) has argued, due to the extreme difficulties present in conceiving an univocal meaning of disease, deciding to privilege one theory over others automatically leads to a revision of at least some of our use of the concept whether we want it to or not (because no theories can fully account for 'disease' as it is now). She goes on to say that the 'only possible justification' for preferring one theory to another has to be one based on pre-existing intuitions about disease rather than normative projections. The tension between these two demands renders the type of definition that is being aimed at impossible. As she explains:

> Presuppositions with respect to what diseases are will always form the basis for building and/or accepting a specific definition. Indeed, one cannot deny that all proposed definitions are based on presuppositions on what is a disease and what not, and hence that an a priori definition on the basis of which one can subsequently decide what is a disease and what not, cannot be given.
>
> (De Vreese, 2016, pp. 6–7)

De Vreese concludes that this impasse will not be overcome by continued use of the methods currently employed. Her main aim in highlighting the deficiencies of contemporary approaches was to encourage others to try new methods and embrace new ways of thinking, somewhat of a theme in this chapter.

Lemoine has also attacked conceptual analysis as an appropriate set of tools for addressing disease. I will examine his ideas in more detail below when I discuss the negative consequences that have been experienced by the field as a whole from pursuing such an approach. But first I will add a further two, broad criticisms.

Epistemic homogeneity and the mental/physical distinction

The first of my two criticisms is that many definitions of disease rely on assumptions about epistemic homogeneity which are not accurate and downplay important aspects of medical conflict, especially in areas where a clear-cut disease concept is supposed to be useful. Because the thinkers in this field are so fixated on the 'what' of disease, there is little space afforded to the 'how' and the 'who'. This is an especially worrying oversight given the fact that who gets to define to disease and how they do it are often the more pressing questions in controversial cases.

The second is that they rely too heavily on being able to easily distinguish between physical and mental illness and do not reflect enough on the difficulty of this distinction. Naturalist positions seem to assume that this division is uncomplicated and that they can focus purely on physiological conditions without having to justify or explain this categorisation. Normativist positions often emphasise the value-laden nature of many psychological diseases, while giving precedence to the role of medical science to identify and legitimise illness. My issue with this is that a biomedical view underlies both positions and as a consequence the theories are unable to adequately explain the many conditions which do not fit neatly into these categories. Contrary to the sharp dichotomy that is often drawn between naturalists and normativists, this is an area where they share many of the same assumptions.

Khushf (2007) has argued strongly for this view. He compared Nordenfelt and Boorse, positioning them as archetype naturalist/normativists, stating that:

> ... both are actually working toward similar ends. Both advance health concepts that seek to tease out fact from value, and reinforce theoretical and social structures that insulate medical science from outside intrusion and distortion. In different ways, both reflect the thought style of modern medicine itself, and both work to preserve its core features.
>
> (Khushf, 2007, p. 20)

He goes on to argue that maintaining a fact/value distinction in our analysis of medicine and disease concepts is likely to become impossible in future, given the material changes to medical infrastructure.[11] But what is important here is his highlighting of assumptions about medical authority, about scientific descriptive ability and about the desire to protect or isolate medicine from the messy value structures of a dynamic and diverse society.

Within this, one of the assumptions that philosophers make when trying to define disease is that there is a workable level of agreement within either medical science (if you are a strict naturalist) or societies as a whole (if you are a normativist) relating to disease states. Without this homogeneity, we would be unable to say that having something deemed undesirable is potentially a disease, because only certain people might think it to be the case. It is true that in many instances, our 'intuitions' about disease are relatively consistent across medical and lay populations, and so comparing some theory of disease against a list of examples like cancer, tuberculosis, typhoid, etc., is straightforward. In these instances, it makes sense to proceed on the basis that there is an uncontroversial set of cases with which to test our ideas. However, there are enough examples where this is not true to make us think twice about this approach.

In these situations, disagreements and discord ring out between doctors, patients and lay individuals. Philosophers of medicine who propose theories of disease bestow upon us with few tools to understand these conflicts. Let us examine a case on the fringes of medical legitimacy to demonstrate what I mean and to bring this discussion back towards contested illnesses.

Morgellons and disease definition

'Morgellons' is a condition that has 'no general medical acceptance as a disease entity' (Mayne et al., 2013). However, it does have symptoms. Primarily, the location of discomfort reported by patients is on, in or under the skin. Individuals complain of painful and frustrating sensations of a stinging, crawling, itching nature. These irritations are accompanied by raw cutaneous lesions which fail over time to heal properly. Alongside these dermatological problems, a host of other issues may be present. Fatigue, joint pain, difficulty remembering words and speaking, headaches and other non-specific symptoms are recorded by patients. Unsurprisingly, perhaps, there is also a high incidence of related conditions that morgellons patients also suffer from including chronic fatigue, depression, obsessive–compulsive disorder (OCD), attention deficit hyperactivity disorder (ADHD), fibromyalgia, joint pain, sleep problems, hair loss and neurological disorders as well as anxiety and substance abuse/dependence (Savely, Leitao and Stricker, 2006; Ahmad and Ramsay, 2009; Hylwa et al., 2012). The number of patients who suffer from

11 Khushf views the clinical/administrative divide as the embodiment of this distinction, and cites recent structural changes to healthcare provision as evidence that the philosophy will likewise have to evolve.

comorbid psychological conditions has been reported as high as 75%. The relationship between these comorbid features is disputed. As is typical with contested illnesses, patients argue that these conditions are symptomatic of morgellons, with doctors more likely to believe that the link between them is correlative.

The most contentious aspects of morgellons is the wrangling between doctors and patients about aetiology and over one symptom in particular. Patients consistently report the existence of protruding material from the skin and blame this for the painful sensations they experience and the sores that develop. Often described as 'fibres' or 'filaments', these 'protruding' items can normally only be viewed through a microscope. Patients have reported these fibres as being of varying length, colour and transparency. This belief is regarded as the 'distinguishing characteristic' of the condition by patients and a small number of researcher advocates.

However, in clinical settings, morgellons sufferers are consistently diagnosed as possessing delusions of parasitosis, an age-old condition that has been recognised for over a century. Delusions of parasitosis (also known as delusional infestation or Ekbom syndrome) is a psychological condition where individuals falsely believe that there are insects, parasites or other unidentified objects about their person and most frequently under their skin which cause them discomfort (Bak et al., 2008; Edlich et al., 2009; Levin and Gieler, 2013). Under this interpretation of morgellons, which is now favoured by the majority of doctors, the open wounds that patients present with are self-inflicted in the process of trying to relieve their symptoms, the fibres in most cases come from clothes and the environment and the comorbid features a function of someone predisposed towards mental illness (Hylwa et al., 2012; Pearson et al., 2012; Freudenmann and Lepping, 2009).[12] In essence, then, according to mainstream medical opinion, morgellons is an old disease dressed up in new clothing. It has been suggested that the alternative disease model which strays from the medical account was galvanised by advances in communications technology, most notably the internet, which allowed patients to converse with each other and form concrete, non-medical aetiological narratives. But also in play here are a group of patients desperate not to be labelled as psychologically ill and extremely adverse to any suggestion that they might be. To them, a psychological diagnosis does nothing but tug the validity of their pain from under their feet.

So, in an instance like this, what are reasonable expectations for a definition of disease? Well, one of the claims made by philosophers is that their ideas may be able to resolve controversial cases by distinguishing disease from non-disease, so perhaps a theory might be able to tell us whether morgellons is a

12 The hardening of medical opinion on the side of a delusional disorder was especially evident following the publication of a CDC report that found no organic signs of pathology.

disease. If we take some of the philosophers we have already examined and apply their ideas to this case, I think it becomes apparent that they possess severe shortcomings. Beginning with Boorse, it is simply unclear as to whether this would be classified as a condition or not. There would seem to be an obvious dysfunction within reference classes, but there is a distinct lack of the kind of biological statistical deviation he is fond of. Though at several points during his work he states that his theory is only applicable to physical illness, he never provides firm demarcation criteria by which to divide the two. He also states that criticisms of his work are only relevant if they refer to 'medically clear cases', which indicates he has little time for the vagaries of something like morgellons. As such, in this instance, it is fairly uncertain as to what his ideas might be able to tell us at all.

Normativist ideas seem more straightforward in this circumstance. Under Cooper's schema, as discussed above, we can see that for a patient, having morgellons would be a bad thing, we would consider that person to be unlucky and their condition would be potentially treatable by medicine. Morgellons, then seems largely unproblematic: it is a disease. Clearly, though, this fails to explain or resolve the enormous controversy surrounding the condition.

If we use some other definitions, we see similar patterns emerge. So, Scadding's (1990) idea of 'biological disadvantage' also renders morgellons a disease because it is true that patients struggle in relationships, their employment prospects are damaged by their condition and their reproductive chances are impaired (his criteria). Wakefield's (1992) influential account defines disorders as 'harmful dysfunctions', and tries to incorporate both a value-laden and factual component into our understanding of the concept (Bolton, 2007). Viewed through the lens of this theory, morgellons would certainly fulfil the 'harmful' portion of the criteria, seeing as it is 'judged negative by sociocultural standards' and 'harmful according to social values'. It is less clear whether it would qualify as a dysfunction, which in this instance is close to Boorse's use of the term. Wakefield (1992, p. 374) describes a dysfunction as a 'scientific and factual term based in evolutionary biology that refers to the failure of an internal mechanism to perform the natural function for which it was designed'. There is not the space here to examine in all its nuances the implications of this definition, but I think it is certainly arguable that morgellons, whether interpreted as a little understood neurological condition, a dermatological concern, a psychological maladjustment or something even more ambiguous, goes some way to fulfilling his criteria.

What these (and other) theories of disease have in common is that they add very little to our understanding of cases like morgellons. There is no space given to the competing interests, the various complicated ways that people feel delegitimised, the alternative aetiologies and why they are believed. Nothing can be extrapolated which might unpick the value disputes present or the power structures which enable them, the way that patients and doctors view disease entities or the heterogeneous responses of individuals and professionals to confusing symptomatic presentation. In short these theories *say* nothing interesting, new or useful about morgellons, or indeed many other conditions that find themselves in the same category. It is not whether morgellons or fibromyalgia or whatever are diseases that is really at stake here, but rather how they are diseases and on whose terms.

In this section I have criticised at length the efforts of various philosophers to define disease in a self-contained manner. I have presented arguments against *any* general theory of disease being successful, by positing that the number of entities hoped to be sufficiently delimited is too great and by putting it that normative theories lack adequate justification. Further to this, I looked at other critiques and raised some questions about that which is left unasked by theories – namely questions about epistemic authority and the true roots of controversy in disease definition. There are, however, more things to say on this topic. Not only do I believe that the literature suffers from major flaws, but that the approach taken by many theorists has unintended consequences of a negative nature on the structure and discourse of the field as a whole. It is at this I will now look.

Consequences of such an approach

It is generally accepted that philosophers working on the disease definition 'problem' are engaging in a form of conceptual analysis (Lemoine, 2013). That is, they are trying to agree upon a cogent definition for a well-known term, as well as uncovering the exact relation between them. In this case, the terms are 'health' and 'disease' as well as, on occasion, 'illness', 'injury', 'disorder', 'dysfunction', etc., though in this section I have focused on 'disease' as a central concern. The method of honing our definitions generally proceeds as follows: a set of uncontroversial examples are treated as foundational, and a list of criteria is drawn up in the form of necessary and sufficient conditions which capture to a great degree these examples. A proponent then argues why their stipulations are the most accurate, anticipates counterexamples and controversial cases and adds any further justifications that they deem relevant. Any opponent wishing to join the conversation must then either attack their definition, propose a new one or do both. I believe that setting up the 'rules of the game' in this manner has a nefarious effect on the sort of philosophy that is produced subsequently.

In this section I will argue that decisions to pursue such an approach limit problem selection and centre the discourse on narrow questions of internal consistency and accurate isomorphism to an agreed set of examples, at the cost of moving the philosophy any closer to practice, patient experience or some other practical measure. The way in which the leading figures in a field conduct their debates colour and direct the rest: it gives a shape and a flavour to the philosophy that others must either replicate or give firm justification as to why they are taking a different path. Most often, they slip into the conversation and follow the established norms, 'having a go' as it were at producing their own definitions to add to the pot.

Lemoine (2013) has argued along these lines, stating that the most influential figures in this field follow the same rough rules, engaging with each other on the basis of fundamental understandings about the kind of theories that would be considered successful. However, this leads to a situation where more than one theory can come to be regarded as reasonably successful and arguments about 'conceptual analyses of "health" and "disease" consist mainly in providing uncontroversial counter-examples to a definition of a term that should successfully account for them' (ibid., p. 316). This is a problem, and it highlights the shortcomings of using conceptual analysis, demonstrating that it is not sufficient in its current form to actually perform the function that is being asked of it: to decide between theories.

Therefore, Lemoine argues, the naturalism/normativism debate will not be resolved in this manner because more than one theorist may feel justified in thinking that they have produced relatively successful definitions of disease and there remains nothing we can reach for that would privilege one account above the other. Worryingly, because of the potential to just keep producing and tweaking theories, this is a situation which left unchecked could continue ad infinitum, albeit in various permutations. His rather devastating pronouncement is that the *only* definitions that conceptual analysis can completely rule out are 'those that nobody would hold, because of some counterintuitive consequence nobody would support'.

Lemoine goes on to argue for a potential way of deciding between naturalism and normativism that goes beyond conceptual analysis, namely calling for the naturalisation of the concept of disease (Lemoine, 2013). However, for our purposes here, his vital contribution is the way in which he so plainly lays out the various internal mechanisms of conceptual analysis in relation to disease definition and demonstrates the ultimately limited usefulness of such an approach. What he picks up on which I would like to expand is the use of counterexamples as a major form of rebuke. I believe that too often the energy expounded by philosophers on the search for a perfect case with which to deliver the knockout blow is a wasted effort. Because though other types of arguments are employed by thinkers, counterexamples are king. However, for the most part, they distract and divert attention from more important matters.

The problem with counterexamples

If you are aiming to refute a theory of disease then there is currently no better way of doing it than to produce an example which quite clearly does not accord with both our intuitive notion of disease and the stipulations provided by your opponent. Luckily for philosophers indulging in this kind of attack, there are so many applicable entities to choose from, both real and potential, that often this is a case of just picking the right one off the shelf to fit your argument. However, this can lead to some bizarre lines of inquiry which, rather than necessarily engaging with the literature in a critically useful way, make the debate entirely about internal logical cogency. Though this doesn't sound like a negative charge, its effect is to drag the discussion further from practice and into ever smaller, ever more irrelevant avenues of discourse. Philosophers consciously operate within a paradigm and their acceptance – sometimes an explicit agreement, sometimes an acquiescence – to the rules of this arrangement is dictating the type of philosophy that gets done.

A good example of this is Rachel Cooper's (2002) discussion of Boorse. She attacks his theory on two fronts, by arguing that his ideas rely on the existence of both natural kinds and clear-cut evolutionary rules of functionality, which, according to her, do not exist in this instance. To support this statement she employs a number of examples. The first of these is actually an extension of an argument used previously by Wright (1973), which is that a Boorsean account of function cannot distinguish accidental from non-accidental contributions to the goal of a system. So, while sweating has the function of cooling down the body and contributing to the goal of regulating body heat, general survival, etc., should you trip and knock a bucket of cold water over yourself that would perform the same role. As we cannot tell the difference between the two, something in Boorse's analysis must be lacking.

To continue with Cooper's critique, her second line of contention is with the notion that it is possible to draw up reference classes in any practical way, which is necessary if we are to define dysfunction in the way Boorse wants us to. Cooper (2002, p. 6–7) argues that due to human variation these would have to be excessively small, in some cases consisting of just one individual, such as 'elderly female Masai mountain-bikers [or] half-Chinese, half-Eskimo boy toddlers'. So as not to single out Rachel Cooper, I will look at some others, for there are many who engage in similar, lengthy discussions of potential shortcomings which can be exposed through clever counterexamples. Lilienfeld and Marino (1995) discuss Wakefield in much the same way. Looking in detail at his theory and focusing on the role that evolution plays in culture, they argue that Wakefield's ideas fail to adequately account for exaptations. In this vein, they put forward criticisms like the following:

> … atheists who are persecuted and ostracised as a result of their beliefs (and thus experience harm) would in many cases be considered disordered according to Wakefield's criteria because, as noted earlier, religious beliefs are probably adaptively neutral exaptations rather than adaptions.
>
> (Lilienfeld and Marino, 1995, p. 413)

What these arguments have in common is their logical accuracy and their practical uselessness. They are both philosophically sound and not fit for purpose. This is because they do not shift the debate in any meaningful way, and continue to point the search-light at component parts of theories rather than the whole beast: the types of theories we produce and the way that we produce them. These criticisms act, in my view, like playful distractions from more important matters – no one outside philosophy considers the function of a bucket of water accidentally spilled to be comparable with sweating, just as nobody believes that atheists who are discriminated against are ill.

A good way of analysing this is to use Illari and Russo's (2014) taxonomy of counterexamples. They compiled a set of counterexamples commonly used by philosophers in debates and ordered them on a spectrum from the broad to the precise. They range in scope from 'all possible worlds' downwards through 'worlds close to the actual world', 'this world', 'some region of this world' to 'some region of this world at some time'. At the broader end of these possible counterexamples, critics can draw upon hypothetical situations from any conceivable environment, as long as they are consistent with the original argument (on the same 'plane' so to speak). Closer to the bottom, counterexamples must be found from the world as it is, some more specific area of the world, or a specific area of the world at a specific time. As may already be clear, the discussions around disease definition currently take place on a 'worlds close to this world' basis, hence the inclusion of elderly female Masai mountain bikers and sufferers of persecuted atheist disease.

I believe that a shift towards something more local would be beneficial, as this would more readily recognise the temporal and contextual nature of all of our philosophical understandings of disease. The way illness is mediated is, I would argue, entirely context dependent, and our philosophical discourse should reflect that.[13] As Floridi (2011, p. 12) has argued in relation to the philosophy of information, trying to generate timeless philosophy does not advance the field because it is 'unable to contribute, keep track of, and interact with, the cultural evolution that philosophical reflection has itself helped to bring about', a statement which could have easily been written about the philosophy of medicine. He argues that philosophy's 'pulling force of innovation has become necessarily external' and again these words ring true, with developments in medical technology, surgical techniques, genetics, the emergence and mutation of previously unknown or unrecognised diseases, and the challenges of an ageing population all serving to inject the philosophy of medicine with intellectual impetus. None of the changes outside of philosophy, as far as I can see, indicate that we should continue down the road of universal theories of disease. If anything, they reassert the diversity, the confusion, the bluster of a world which cannot be simplified and bent into the confines of stipulation. Without true acknowledgement of the criticisms I

13 This is *not* the same as saying I think that disease itself – however you wish to bracket it – is somehow context dependent, or that diseases are constructions of society. Rather it is the way that we understand disease, and indeed what we understand *to be* disease, which is grounded in a here and now or there and then.

have laid out here, philosophy of medicine – Caplan's 'intellectual island' – will edge ever closer to disappearing off the horizon, unable to speak for, to, or about pressing issues in modern medicine.

There is, however, another aspect of contemporary philosophy of medicine that is, on the face of it at least, engaging more actively with practice and patients. This is the phenomenology of illness, a topic that I feel deserves a few words now.

The phenomenology of illness

The branch of philosophy known as phenomenology is instructive here for several reasons.[14] Firstly, it has directed the 'problem of disease' away from a concern of demarcation and towards a set of broader questions, such as how philosophy might and ought to respond to illness, and in what ways philosophy might be useful to the sick themselves and those around them. Secondly, it weaves ancient and contemporary thought together in the same framework, using illness to inform long-standing and central philosophical questions. Thirdly, and most importantly here, phenomenologists working on disease do what I have criticised others for not doing: they engage with medicine, with patients and with sickness in a manner that is not only illuminative but also has potentially practical consequences.

Havi Carel (2016a), a prominent phenomenologist, makes the claim that illness is a '*violent invitation* to philosophise' (emphasis in original) because of the way it compromises the normal subject–object operation of embodied selfhood and makes us confront our bodily existence, whether we would like to do so or not. Illness, in this sense an interruption, an uninvited disjuncture, forces us to approach our embodied selves in a new way.

This focus on embodiment and being-in-the-world has many benefits. It not only gives us tools and insights to challenge the Cartesian spirit so present in both medical and lay understandings of the body but it also exposes the extensive reach and fault-lines of such a worldview. Furthermore, this work focuses on the experience of disease in a way that other philosophy avoids: it is messy, subjective, narrative, qualitative. But is it also, I believe, edifying. Unlike the high-minded conceptual tussles described in this chapter, phenomenology offers patients a way of approaching their condition that may allow them to achieve 'wellbeing within illness', while at the same time reminding doctors that the biomedical world they describe to a patient may not be isomorphic with the sufferer's experience (Carel, 2007).

14 I do not have the space here for a discussion of what the phenomenological method *is*, or to describe the various intellectual currents within the field. For canonical texts, see Husserl (2012), Merleau-Ponty (2013), Sartre (1969) and Heidegger (1978). For an overview, see Moran (1999).

Though most of the 20th-century thinkers who loom large over phenomenology – Heidegger, Merleau-Ponty, Husserl – had little specific to say about illness, they bestowed upon later writers a sophisticated method for approaching the problem. It is these thinkers I will briefly examine here, from the work of S. Kay Toombs and Drew Leder through to more recent studies by Havi Carel (for an overview, see Carel, 2016b). Taken together, their body of work appears to represent a serious challenge to reductionist models of medicine and draws attention to both the transformative and informative nature of disease as an subject of inquiry.

S. Kay Toombs, a philosopher with multiple sclerosis, has written extensively and originally on the phenomenology of illness. Ironically, given the critique provided above, her starting point is that there are essential (Toombs terms them 'eidetic') features to the illness experience, not specific to one condition (though it should be noted she later weakened this position, refashioning 'essential' features as 'typical': Toombs, 1993). These characteristics, which 'transcend the peculiarities and particularities of different disease states and constitute the meaning of illness-as-lived', revolve around loss: the loss of certainty, of control, of freedom to act, of the familiar world and of a sense of wholeness (Toombs, 1987).

These aspects of illness are common and universal, she argues, but her intention is not to bracket 'illness' as a category to be delineated or denied in the manner of disease. Rather, she hopes to show how the 'world' of illness and the patient – whose spatial and temporal structure fluctuates – is separate from that of the physician, who deals in the body-as-object and the disease-as-entity, and suggests that a greater understanding of these disparities would pave the way for better care.[15] Patients and doctors need to work together to find a shared language, recognising that the manner in which one party (those who are ill) experience illness not as a biological dysfunction but as a rupture of their lived body dictates what are and are not appropriate forms of communication.

Bringing prolonged attention to the ways in which disease alters our experience of the world, and to the consequences of these changes, was, in my view, Toombs's key contribution.[16] She outlined the ways in which disease is capable of rendering the world a changed place, in which objects with previously unambiguous and benign roles now appear to be obstacles or challenges. Furthermore, she described the alienation that can arise when a patient and a physician talk past each other, one about normal ranges and white blood cell counts, the other about not being able to walk up the hill to their house. Ultimately, it is this that Toombs was trying to make us understand: that serious

15 I have simplified this account in the interests of brevity – following on from Sartre, Toombs actually identifies four layers of illness experience (Toombs, 1990; Toombs, 1993).

16 This insight was not limited to disease, but also applied to disability (Toombs, 1995).

disease is almost always transformative, and by interpreting that transformation in narrow biomedical terms, we run the risk of witnessing successful communication between doctor and patient break down. Patients and physicians must not let their different experiences of the same body (the body-as-lived and the body-as-analysed) mean that total delineation occurs, and neither finds themselves speaking to the other about the same thing.

Other writers have used phenomenology and personal experience to make broader points about the metaphysical scaffolds that support our world views (or 'habits of mind', in the language of some phenomenologists). For example, in *The Absent Body*, his masterful study of embodiment, Drew Leder (1990) utilises an intense examination of our bodies as experienced (or not) in order to highlight not just what is taken for granted about our everyday bodily lives but also to undermine the tendency towards disembodiment which he takes to lie beneath our entire intellectual tradition. He does this by first explicating in detail the way in which our bodies are often removed from consciousness, whether obscured, forgotten, automated or otherwise concealed from our attention. It is difficult, he says, to become aware of a body so often relegated in this manner. 'Feelings of general neutrality', he writes (Leder, 1990, p. 72), 'or well-being are typically amorphous, marked neither by definable beginnings and ends nor abrupt transformations.' A large part of his study focuses on the ways in which this 'invisibility' occurs, and the interruption that disease causes to such an arrangement, but the most important contribution he makes, as far as this discussion goes, is his unrelenting assault on the clean division of mind and body, a process of disembodiment he views as 'an abiding stream in Western intellectual history'.

The problem he identifies and criticises is the way in which our medical notions of embodiment are based upon abstractions or, when they are tied to the flesh, upon a mechanistic thematisation of corpses. As he says:

> We can inspect a dead body in a way we cannot the living. Modern medicine, profoundly Cartesian in spirit, has contrived to use the corpse as a methodological tool and a regulative ideal. Medical education begins with the cadaver, just as the clinical case ends with the pathoanatomical dissection. Death unveils the truths of the inner body and its diseases … Notions of embodiment based upon the corpse can lead to an objectivist, depersonalised medicine. The physician need not attend to the patient's intentionality when he or she is conceived of as a physiological machine.
> (Leder, 1990, pp. 146–147)

Though Foucault, Bishop and overs have covered similar ground, as discussed previously, Leder makes an interesting point which I would like to touch upon. He argues that a positive feedback loop exists between dualist metaphysics and western society, a process that gets experienced on a bodily level. In other words, what began as a theoretical abstraction has become codified into ways of seeing and organising the world, which in turn feeds back into and strengthens our dualistic schematisations of our bodies and disease. 'We are all to some extent Cartesians', he writes (ibid., p. 108), 'either willingly or struggling to get free'.

I think there is something profoundly correct about this, though it can express itself in oblique ways. Patients find, as will be discussed in the second half of this book, that they simply do not have the language to adequately describe what is happening to them. This is because of a fundamental failure of categorisation – the prevailing notion that the phenomenological world can be neatly assimilated into the biomedical one. That this assimilation does not happen, or happens in a clumsy, inelegant way, is no surprise, but this does not lessen the negative effects of such a failed integration. What Leder points to – what I am pointing to – is the sense that our entire system of categorisation is flawed, and that it cannot encompass that which we think it can or should.

Havi Carel is a contemporary philosopher who has written extensively on the phenomenology of illness, covering too broad a range of topics to be effectively summarised here.[17] In place of an overview I would like instead to mention two particular components of her work: her repeated assertion that illness is a fantastically apt subject for philosophers to work on and her attempts to use philosophical tools in a wide variety of circumstances. The questions she asks as a result of this approach are more direct, more personal, more relevant. Can we, for example, be happy within illness? What can philosophy teach us about being sick and can it change our experience of sickness for the better? A person with chronic illness herself, she writes:

> I have the most pressing and personal interest in understanding the illness experience and in thinking about how to make that experience less lonely, alienated and socially scripted. In the years since I was diagnosed I have navigated my rickety boat of selfhood between the Scylla of medicalisation and objectification of my illness and Charybdis of social pressures to conform to the ideal of 'the good patient' or 'sick role'. When subjected to philosophical analysis, this navigation, both philosophically salient and pragmatically important, can help us understand illness as part of selfhood: it is thus of prime philosophical value.
>
> (Carel, 2016c, p. 582)

What she touches on here is something I wish to echo: severe illness is a philosophically fascinating and serious object of inquiry, the grip of which only

17 For example, she extends Toombs's thoughts about the losses that illness can bring, focusing in particular on the loss of freedom, discusses the ways in which illness can have a benign effect on a person's wellbeing or at least provoke a surprisingly positive reaction (see also Kidd, 2012), expands Fricker's notion of epistemic injustice and also provides several in-depth, phenomenological accounts of breathlessness as part of a large, collaborative project called 'Life of Breath'.

the luckiest of us are likely to completely escape. It makes us think about ourselves, about our limitations and our strengths, it puts enough strain on our relationships to show them for what they are; it brings us closer to death, whether that entails reflection, contentment, fear or something else; it removes us from the sanitised world we have created and reminds us of our biology, while pushing us into the hands of expensive, gleaming pieces of technology. It is transformative, in other words, though the nature of the transformation is unpredictable and idiosyncratic. Disease affects everyone in different ways:

> The values and desires of ill people can alter. They may slow down or speed up, reconsider their career, or want to spend more time with their family; they might find new meaning in work or as a volunteer, and they may value time and simply living in the present more highly. Goals and ambitions are often updated, taking into account the limitations and opportunities brought about by illness, perhaps becoming more focused on what is still possible. Their world-view may change deeply. They may become depressed, or more religious, or happier. And, of course, they may not change at all.
>
> (Carel, Kidd and Pettigrew, 2016, p. 1153)

I stated at the beginning of this brief section that the work of phenomenologists has practical consequences, and I do believe this to be true. I think it could be of great comfort to an individual to come to see their condition not simply as an unwanted, external intrusion into their lives but as something that transfigures their way of being, this transfiguration not being by necessity a negative or wholly negative experience. Likewise, I think it could be of great help to a physician to more deeply understand that the world they transpose from textbooks onto their patients is not the same world that the individual in their clinic lives in. But, having stated these positions as I have, does it not seem fairly self-evident that illness is transformative and that doctors should think about things from the perspective of the patient? And, undoubtedly useful as philosophy might be to some individuals in coming to terms with their new position in life, so might self-help books, or running, or listening to Radio 3.

Phenomenology, however, is not so glib.[18] Having accounts of illness like Carel's and Toombs's (or others, like Paul, 2014), which peg themselves closely to the patient experience in all its permutations allows us to consider illness in a fuller, more complete manner – it gives us more to chew on, so to speak.

It is also complimentary to much work that has been completed in the sociology of health and illness, and works in tandem with it by providing a philosophical explication of the personal level of meaning and interaction to

18 I mean by this that it is glib to say that illness transforms. How it does so, in what way and for what reason – these are the real questions.

supplement the social. A good example of this is how Toombs's concepts of the patient's and doctor's separate 'worlds' compliments Mishler's (1984) idea of the lifeworld: Toombs provides an experiential account of the broken interactional model that Mishler famously described by analysing doctor-patient transcripts.

Phenomenology thus reinforces what sociologists have been arguing for decades: patients' views matter, disease is not best understood solely as a biological dysfunction, illness alters the functional boundaries of an individual's life. But it also utilises sophisticated philosophical tools to challenge biomedicine, highlight epistemic injustice and recognise all the ways in which disease is 'world-changing'. Phenomenology sets itself apart from other aspects of philosophy of medicine by being attentive to disease as it is lived, by being conceptually astute and by offering deep analysis of the breakdowns that occur along common fault lines. However, that does not mean that it is perfect.

The problem with phenomenology

As has been noted, phenomenologists of illness often position their work as a challenge to naturalist theories of disease, and believe their embodied, spatio-temporal analysis to produce a more humanistic, true-to-life vision of illness, while simultaneously acting as both a guide to patients and doctors on how the experience of disease and healthcare can be mediated more successfully. However, the nature of this positioning, and the objects against which phenomenology are supposedly arranged, begin to appear suspect upon deeper consideration.

Precisely what is the relationship between phenomenologists and the other segments of philosophy of disease discussed above? It has been noted that most frequently, phenomenologists talk about their work as it relates to naturalism, or what they regard to be naturalism. Carel (2008), for example, has stated that her account of illness is meant to 'augment' naturalist theories of disease; Svenaeus (2017), another prominent phenomenologist of illness, goes further, describing his philosophy as a consciously 'anti-naturalistic' body of work. The overall sense, reading phenomenologists, is that they *disapprove* of naturalism (in the words of Ferry-Danini, 2018, they are 'wary' of it), and feel that phenomenology adds depth to our understanding of disease by fleshing out aspects of being ill not adequately accounted for otherwise. That is to say, they believe that naturalistic viewpoints do not allow us to understand disease in anything but a supremely restricted manner which, lacking the adjunctive input of phenomenology, prevents us from seeing the full picture.

However, as has been argued by Ferry-Danini (2018) and Sholl (2015), phenomenologists seem willingly confused as to the exact nature of the viewpoint they are criticising, unaware of the ways in which their work compliments (and in fact, with its rigid disease/illness demarcation, reinforces) rather than challenges it, and overly prone to simplifying oppositional standpoints. It is also suggested that phenomenologists conflate medical science, healthcare provision and very specific instances of doctor patient interaction, meshing them together as 'medicine'. In short: who and what are actually their target? What empirical evidence can they provide for the apparent claims they make in stacking the deck as they do (i.e. that most doctors are naturalists, that medical care is reductionist the majority of the time)? And in what sense does phenomenology *challenge* this rather than act as the descriptive half of a disease/illness dichotomy?

What emerges from this critique is that phenomenologists are want to regard naturalism, if not explicitly, as a by-word for *ontological* naturalism, in that their criticisms seem to revolve around the epistemic privileging of naturalistic explanations or, in some cases, their apparent total domination of any kind of meaning-making around disease and illness. This is, unfortunately, something of a straw man. Naturalist explanations, even at the Boorsean end of things, leave room for a non-scientific, illness dimension – that is to say they demarcate disease as being scientifically determined but accept that this is then given certification by its life in the social world (hence why homosexuality or periodontal disease are not regarded as illnesses). Furthermore, *within* a purely naturalistic framework, a multitude of non-reductionist viewpoints proliferate as Sholl writes:

> It is perfectly naturalistic to describe human beings as complex, multidimensional, and dynamic as a result of their biological plasticity and ability to shape their environment. While some have tried to redefine health and disease based on the biological property of homeostasis, an even more dynamic understanding of how humans adapt to and anticipate environmental stressors can be seen in the concept of allostasis, which describes how humans and other organisms change biochemically, physiologically, and even behaviourally to meet varying internal and external demands.
>
> (Sholl, 2015, p. 398)

Overall then, and I would agree, it is hard to regard phenomenology as a legitimate, wholesale alternative to the approaches I detailed at the start of this chapter. Having said that, I am of a mind to be charitable with regard to phenomenology, and I think it can make a valuable contribution to our understanding of disease. Where I believe the real issue to arise between phenomenologists and naturalism is not on the higher-level, theoretical plain where much philosophy gets discussed, but rather the sense that phenomenologists have – often as patients more than philosophers – that their and others' experience is being read, not to mention interrogated, in a naturalistic way. What I mean by this is that phenomenologists recognise the tension between the embodied, 'world-changing' nature of disease and the unsatisfactory *expressions* of naturalism – whether it be the medical gaze, pharmaceutical responses to complex issues, a doctor speaking past you – that seem to permeate a lot of medical encounters (and, indeed, interactions with lay people), regardless of the actual permutations of theoretical naturalism. This is a generous view, given the critique, but I feel that it holds: phenomenology is a reaction not so much to other philosophy as to real life, a life full of experiences which confirm that *whether or not* medicine reduces disease to an irresponsible degree theoretically, it can certainly feel like that. And if you come from a tradition in which experiential epistemology is your primary epistemology, it is then of little surprise that these kinds of viewpoints are pushed front and centre.

Before I conclude this chapter, I would like briefly to pick up one further strand in the philosophy of disease, that of the French philosopher Georges Canguilhem.

Canguilhem

Georges Canguilhem was a totemic thinker in the history and philosophy of science. One of the key questions he grappled with related to the study of biology and the distinction between the mechanistic logic of experimental epistemology and the inherent variability of life: how can we study biological entities in full when the methods we employ demand of them things that they are not? In other words, the tools we possess for generating knowledge about living beings are predicated on the objects of study being inert systems, manipulatable and constant. Life, on the other hand, as Canguilhem understands it, is resistant to these techniques of analysis because it is relational and interactive, something that becomes clearest in his views on physiology and medicine. It 'disconcerts logic' (Canguilhem, 1991, p. 1) in its capacity to exist across a multitude of norms, dependent on its environment, and its dynamic ability to change in the face of new conditions. As he says:

> What characterises health is a capacity to tolerate variations in norms on which only the stability of situations and milieus – seemingly guaranteed yet in fact always necessarily precarious – confers a deceptive value of definitive normality. Man is truly healthy only when he is capable of several norms, when he is more than normal. The measure of health is a certain capacity to overcome organic crises and to establish a new physiological order, different from the old. Health is the luxury of being able to fall ill and recover. Every disease is, by contrast, a reduction of the power to overcome others.
>
> (Canguilhem, 2008, p. 132)

For Canguilhem, it makes no sense to talk of organs or cells being diseased or pathological, because his conceptual ideas are contextual; health and disease are characterised as a disposition towards changing circumstances, an ability to cope or not cope with new environments. They are also evaluative, in that he believed any distinctions drawn between 'the normal and the pathological' to be qualitative judgements rather than quantitative absolutes; 'normal' is not the opposite of 'diseased', because the diseased body is simply a body living according to new and different norms.

Though there is far more that could be said here, and though Canguilhem's relationship to vitalism, physiology and biology more generally (not to mention 20th-century French politics, phenomenology and Foucault) is fascinating, I will try to tie what has been said to the discussion being had in this book. It is immediately clear that whatever his respect for (and close attention to) biology, he is no naturalist. Diseases are not mechanical malfunctions of the body, or statistical deviations of its systems, and his point is that life cannot be fully accounted for in this way (Canguilhem, 2008). Furthermore, he strove to demonstrate that the statistically frequent is not necessarily normal and that it would likewise be a mistake to conflate the statistically infrequent with the pathological; as such, his analysis would have little time for Boorse and other's attempts to cleave the body's systems into healthy and diseased ranges, even within the limited contextualisation of reference classes (Spicker, 1987).

Neither, though, is he a normativist, at least in the sense outlined in the first part of this chapter. He does take health and disease to be evaluative concepts, but not in the same way that normativists do. The normativism in Canguilhem's work, if that is what you want to call it, is individuated rather than universal, dynamic rather than static: a person might feel well and be happy, while at the same time exist perilously between states of ill-health, existing in a narrow (for them) habitable zone, while another may feel sick but be capable of tolerating rapidly changing conditions. It is the interaction between these two levels, the phenomenological experiences of illness and the inter- and intra-relational ability of a particular body to withstand the changing of norms within itself and its environment, that mean Canguilhem's conception of disease transcends the naturalist–normativist divide.

The insight he might offer our analysis of contested illness is difficult to discern, given the close attention he paid to the biological markers of disease and their conspicuous absence in these cases. That being said, it is clear that his complex view of sickness as being in some definitive way related to the adaptability of persons to new milieus is instructive here: the contested illness patient's subjective experience of their environment is marked by a deterioration in function, and whether this interactional conflict is founded upon something viral, bacterial or indeed traumatic or emotional, is of less relevance than the fact that the symptoms experienced by patients arise somehow from this situational context and contract and diminish the patient's ability to adapt to new norms of life. In fact, as we shall see when we examine fibromyalgia in more detail, it is precisely the inability of many patients to adapt, psychologically, to the new circumstances fostered upon them by illness that sets them apart from other sets of patients, this observation folding in on itself when we wonder whether the thing that is driving such mental incompatibility with illness and the illness itself are one and the same thing.

Towards a philosophy of contested disease

This chapter has been a critical analysis of the way that, over a number of years, certain strands of philosophy have approached the problem of disease. I have noted the motivations, both potential and given, for this undertaking and found that the aims of theorists are insufficiently fulfilled by their attempts. What's more, it seems highly likely, as detailed here, that it is not the attempts themselves that are the root cause of this failure but in many cases the method by which they are assembled in the first place. Of particular relevance to this thesis is the lack of contribution such theories make to our understanding of contested illnesses. Many of the issues I detailed in the first chapter are at most lightly brushed by the ideas discussed here. But if we are to insert philosophy into these problems (and I think we must), then where to begin?

Focus, certainly: diseases not disease. A continued acknowledgement of the complicated and the inexplicable and the diverse; a tendency to shy away from attempted containment, universalism and essentialism, instead falling more towards individuated experience. A desire too, whether in analysis or description, to imagine other worlds, other ways of being patients, of being doctors, of being bodies, this being in itself the surest method to avoid acceding total epistemic stewardship to medical science, remembering always that we are not simply engaging with a scientific enterprise but with a process inseparably tied up with symbolic meaning. It is this – the production and dissemination of meaning – that philosophers of medicine should be most concerned with, and yet it is a subject on which many remain largely tight-lipped. What do we think, why do we think it, how does it affect our health and can we shift our perceptions to make us feel better? These are more useful questions.

As Timmermans and Haas (2008) convincingly argued (in relation to sociology, but their critique might likewise apply to philosophy), thinkers can too often be detached from the medical fleshiness of their subjects, making straw men of reductionist healthcare, conflating different diseases, or the same diseases across different populations, or the same diseases in different stages of development, and ignoring the intricate and relevant feedback loops between disease, healthcare, identity and outcomes. As I argued previously, what is at play here is the separation of interest between disease and illness, a disciplinary distinction most often found in sociology which is happy on the one hand to afford medical science epistemic control over disease while on the other to regularly criticise the results of such control, as viewed through the prism of unhappy illness experiences. Philosophers are little better in their bracketing.

Fundamentally, however, the philosophy of medicine literature around disease frustrates because of the lack of insight it offers into people's lives. This may be too lofty an aim to bestow upon what is, really, an intellectual exercise much like many others, but disease appears to me to be a particular topic of inquiry that, more than invites, *demands* serious reflection. It is the imposition of an altered state on a person, for sure, but it is also the meeting place of biology, culture, science, technology and economics. Contested illnesses, to as much if not greater degree so than other diseases, sit at such junctions, and their study tells us so much more than simply a reductive narrative of personal impairment.

A focus on the particulars of a disease or disease state raises the status of philosophical patient-hood too, especially at the stranger, more controversial end of things. It has a humanising function. A sick individual moves from abstractly possessing a counterexample to embodying a universal truth rendered specific by culture, time, place and person.

Fibromyalgia patients, confronted with a state of being in which constant pain appears to be an emergent property, coalesced indeterminately from the moving parts of their lives, cannot be explicated along virtually any of the axes that might give their experience or their condition meaning using the tools that philosophy of disease grants us; the political and personal complexities that swirl around contested illnesses such as this are elided by a philosophical view of disease that attempts to flatten the human experience – either by acting as though it is of no consequence, as naturalists do, or by assigning to it a homogeneity and simplicity it has never and will never possess. The philosophy discussed at the beginning of this chapter has one thing in common: it renders the problematic unproblematic, and disease is always problematic. As Canguilhem writes, disease is only given life in individuated circumstances at the level of the organism – it must touch us socially and psychologically, on this higher level, to be considered illness at all:

> In the final analysis, would it not be appropriate to say that the pathological can be distinguished as such, that is, as an alteration of the normal state, only at the level of organic totality, and when it concerns man, at the level of conscious individual totality, where disease becomes a kind of evil?
>
> (Canguilhem, 1991, p. 44)

Chapter 4

Shorter, Showalter, Hacking

Introduction

In the previous chapter, I discussed the relevance (or lack thereof) that contemporary philosophy of medicine has to the question of contested illness. That question, or rather cluster of questions, being in some strong sense to do with the way we experience illness, both as patients and as healthy bystanders; those questions essentially being:

- What qualifies instinctively as disease and how does it do so?
- What do we expect to look at when we look at a sick person?
- How do we assimilate, reject or mediate information given to us by our bodies, by professionals and by the people around us?
- What are the social and institutional contexts in which these diseases live?

We may not, indeed, be much closer to answering these concerns, but I have begun to sketch out the foundations of the discussion. Legitimacy, validation, responsibility, biomedicine, embodiment – all these find a place in our language of disease, and in particular of contested disease. By the end of this chapter I will have added a handful more. And although I believe there is little to be usefully gleaned from the disease definition debate in terms of helping us to understand the philosophical underpinnings of contested illnesses, this does not mean that no interesting or relevant scholarly work has been completed which can further our comprehension of what is, at its most clear, a muddied subject.

In this chapter, I will turn my attention to two historians and a philosopher who in many ways could also be classified as a historian. The former pair, Edward Shorter and Elaine Showalter, have both courted controversy in patient communities with their historical analysis of psychosomatic illnesses, psychiatry and, in the case of Showalter, hysteria specifically. The reasons for this are, I surmise, a combination of form and content. Their theses, though distinct, overlap in many significant ways: they believe that chronic fatigue syndrome, fibromyalgia and many other similar conditions exist on a historical continuum with previous psychosomatic conditions, and that they are for all intents and purposes the current incarnation of hysteria. That is to say, of emotional distress finding an outlet subconsciously through physical symptoms, the exact manifestation of which is dependent on prevailing notions of acceptability. This does not sit well with those who believe their illness to be primarily organic and whose identity has come to a certain extent to be formed in opposition to those who say or act as though it isn't. Both writers present this idea in a forthright manner, which does not endear them to patient communities who feel belittled and patronised. It is, however, notable that while they remain controversial figures for many individuals with contested illnesses, they have received minimal criticism from fellow academics.[1]

It is my intention to give the ideas presented by Shorter and Showalter a fair reading and to analyse the claims they make, especially relating to subconscious symptom selection (drawn from the so-called 'symptom pool'), cultural transmission of disease and how the changing nature of the doctor–patient relationship and the family have affected patients. The last of the three, Ian Hacking, is a philosopher who has written extensively about dynamic nominalism and the relationship between individuals and the categories they are placed (or place themselves) into. His exemplary studies of multiple personality disorder and dissociative fugue are the brightest stars in a constellation of writings around this topic and though his work follows in the long tradition of natural kinds, the ways in which he has adapted nominalist debates into a modern framework of interaction – positioning himself between a Foucauldian structural analysis and Goffman's closely observed sociology of mental illness – give it resonance for the discussion here. Principally, Hacking's ideas concern identity and the structure of thought, memory and identity, and their relation to contested illness will be examined in the second half of this book.

What all three of these writers have in common is the importance they place on viewing patients in context. A sick person is never just a sick person. They are part of a group of individuals experiencing similar sensations, part of a society that gently and not-so-gently nudges them towards certain patterns of behaviour and explanation and away from others, and in the process they become both willing and non-willing, conscious and unconscious agents of their own distress. That this happens is, to some extent, less contentious or problematic than how it happens. How do shady interactions with the vagaries of 'culture' produce specific illness behaviour and beliefs? Is the restructuring of experience that is posited to occur anything close to a consistent process?

That questions like these lie at the heart of the work discussed below is in large part why I have chosen to discuss it in the first place. There would be a

1 For an example of the backlash against Shorter, see Scott and Scott (2003). For a description of the reaction to Showalter, see Larkin (1998).

great deal missing from our understanding of disease and contested diseases if we were to lean solely on the philosophy of disease literature for analytic support, and so by bringing in these thinkers from other disciplines, I hope to cast more light and shadow on the topic at hand.

Shorter

Edward Shorter has been described as a 'highly critical' historian of psychosomatic conditions (Hacking, 1998, p. 158). There are four strands of his work that are relevant here: the historical continuity of past psychosomatic conditions with modern illnesses, the subconscious mind's desire to be respected and to choose ways of expressing its pain that reflect this, the decline in trust between doctor and patient and the increased atomisation and loneliness of postmodern family life. Taken together, these provide a coherent if conservative explanation and analysis of contested illnesses, and one which makes us question the consequences of sympathetic doctors, the role of the media and indeed the entire social matrix of the modern patient.

Historical continuity

Across his two most famous works on the subject, *From Paralysis to Fatigue* and *From the Mind into the Body*, Shorter argues strongly for a total historical continuity between hysteria, railway spine, shellshock, neurasthenia and any number of other ancient appellations for unexplained medical symptoms with conditions we see around us today such as chronic fatigue, Gulf War syndrome and fibromyalgia (Shorter, 1993; Shorter, 1994). That is not to say that a fibromyalgia patient feels and presents in the same way as a hysteric, just that the root cause is the same. Shorter believes that undulations in the professional structure of medicine and psychiatry, as well as various ripples across the cultural life of the societies in question, lead in some slippery but tangible way to different symptoms being 'popular' at different times.[2] The conditions *are* different, then, in the sense that the way patients present in clinics changes as you look over the years. However, this metamorphosis of symptomatic profile forms a large part of Shorter's evidence, for he contends that our body only expresses emotional disquiet in ways which are considered acceptable and explicable in the social and intellectual milieu in which it exists.

Paralysis, then, as an example, was 'a culturally specific nineteenth century mode of processing extreme emotion' and is not seen today in as great

2 I put 'popular' inside quotation marks because although Shorter frequently employs this kind of adjective, along with 'fashionable', 'trendy' and the like, I find that the connotations of conscious decision-making and glibness associated with these words detract from their relevance as descriptors. I am not the only one to think Shorter's loose relationship with language can undermine his scholarship – Fitzhugh Mullan makes a similar point (Mullan, 1986).

numbers because it is not as deeply imbedded into our social consciousness as a way of experiencing distress legitimately. This can be observed in the way that, while once common among a certain class of young women, paralysis ceases to be seen frequently once the Babinski sign and test became well known: it is difficult to claim you are paralysed when an 'objective' test of your reflexes finds them to be working normally. The same could be said for claiming to have a strange object or animal inside you once the power of X-rays became well disseminated or for professing issues with your heart, lungs or sensory organs after these became exceptionally easy to monitor and investigate with the tools and feelers of modern medicine. The argument goes that once paralysis (or whatever) becomes somehow discredited or illegitimate, the body will find another, more acceptable or, at least, less disprovable, way of somatising.

Shorter is clearly very much of the opinion that while there is something permanent about 'organic' conditions, or diseases with an identifiable physical lesion, psychosomatic illnesses, both then and now, are permanent only in their cause and vary wildly in their manifestation. That this cause itself is vague – a sort of maladjustment, an unrealised discontent – only serves to make them more difficult to identify and analyse. The specific symbolism of this unhappiness may migrate from one vector to another; the nineteenth century woman unknowingly reacting against the stupefying passivity that defined her femininity is different from the man returning from the trenches was unable to reconcile his apparently civilised day-to-day life with the horror he witnessed, but both are uniform in the sense that they are unhappy in ways they do not comprehend. What Shorter says is that to these archetypes we can add the career-driven yuppies of the 1980s who suddenly found themselves unimaginably tired and lonely divorcees wrestling with an unfulfilling and tedious existence who begin to ache all over.[3] Their cultural and personal situation is different and thus the symptoms they experience are not the same, but the heart of the problem remains that their bodies are expressing sadness without informing their minds. Or rather, that this is their method of informing them.

What is evident from the outset is that Shorter is keen to dispel concerns of insensitivity and is worried about being misunderstood. On the very first page of *From Paralysis to Fatigue* he states:

> It should be emphasised … that from the patient's viewpoint psychosomatic problems qualify as genuine diseases. There is nothing imaginary or simulated about the patient's perception of his or her illness. Although the symptom may be psychogenic, the pain or grinding fatigue is very real.
>
> (Shorter, 1993, p. ix)

3 Shorter notes that a diagnosis of hysteria or similar is as likely to emerge from a life of leisure as it is from extreme hardship (Shorter, 1994, p. 66).

His lip-service to the reality of the pain is undermined however, by repeatedly implying throughout his work that psychogenic mechanisms are ontologically less valid than biological ones. By arguing that, in one case, organic disease, both symptoms and internal distress are 'real', while maintaining that only half of this duality is present in a somatiser, he drives a wedge between them that privileges organic illness. At no point does he adequately examine or explain why the metaphysical basis for one form of reality (pain caused by an anatomically observable dysfunction), is placed above another (pain caused by some other, harder to identify mechanism, as with psychogenesis).

For Shorter, physical diseases are the permanent or semi-permanent bedfellows of mankind. They are constant throughout history.[4] Psychosomatic conditions, on the other hand, are products of a time and place, morally charged in a way that other diseases aren't, and heavily, heavily influenced by outside factors.[5] What are these outside factors? Shorter speaks often of the 'symptom pool', which we will turn to now.

The symptom pool

To display 'acceptable' symptoms, as used by Shorter (1993, p. x), is to perform sickness in a way that absolves moral responsibility for your illness, but also in a way that accords with the expectations and prevailing scientific notions of biological illness behaviour:

> The unconscious mind, just like the conscious, is influenced by surrounding culture, which has models of what it considers to be legitimate and illegitimate symptoms. Legitimate symptoms are ascribed to an underlying organic disease for which the patient could not possibly be blamed. Illegitimate ones, by contrast, may be thought due to playacting or silliness. By defining certain symptoms as illegitimate, a culture strongly encourages patients not to develop them or risk being thought 'undeserving' individuals with no real medical problems. Accordingly there is a great pressure on the unconscious mind to produce only

4 This seems a contentious claim. It does not seem unreasonable to argue that to a (perhaps lesser) degree what Shorter considers 'organic' disease is also greatly affected by its social surroundings. Plenty of conditions require specific environments in order to flourish and come and go historically – for example water-borne diseases in heavily populated areas. Furthermore, some diseases simply *are* different: to take a common example, the diabetes patient of today would be unrecognisable to doctors even in the mid-20th century (see Polonsky, 2012).

5 It should be noted he is talking about symptomatic presentation here, with a consistent underlying mechanism. As he writes, '[the] tendency to convert unhappiness into physical symptoms is probably universal in the human species' (Shorter, 1994, p. 88).

> legitimate symptoms ... the unconscious mind desires to be taken seriously and not be ridiculed.
>
> (Shorter, 1993, p. x)

There are three identifiable parts to what Shorter would consider a legitimate symptom. It must accord with overriding ideas of validity, that is to say that for a symptom to be acceptable it should relate to some current theory or other of the body that is widely acknowledged to be correct. This idea can then be used to explain how symptoms have changed over time in tandem with movements in general aetiological frameworks of disease. The second part is intertwined with the first, that the symptoms displayed must work to absolve the patient of moral responsibility for their illness. This is usually most successfully achieved by mimicking that which has the most credence and commands the most respect, and in this cultural context that means established, observable, quantifiable, organic disease.[6] The third part of this idea, by implication, is that there exists some powerful mechanism of cultural transference which imbues in the popular mind a list of acceptable and non-acceptable means of being ill, which in times of crisis is used to communicate emotional dysfunction in a painful physical language.

Shorter suggests two further clarifications of this point. Firstly, he puts emphasis on the doctor–patient relationship as a means by which sick individuals are able to gauge what is expected of their bodies according to the ideas of the day. He does not place this inside a simplistic framework of suggestion, Charcot-style, but provides a more sophisticated account of an important dynamic which has changed over time from one of idolatry and patriarchal hierarchy to a process based more on individualistic market models of health-care, growing mistrust of authority and a preference for pharmaceuticals.

Secondly, he argues that patients are aware or become aware of the 'trends' in symptomatic presentation which are most in harmony with contemporary explanations of illness. How this occurs has likewise developed over time, from the popular culture of the nineteenth century, be it novels, the theatre or forms of spa tourism, to the sensationalist mass media and day-time talk shows of the 1990s, and on to our own era of truly instant, mass communication, all the while buffeted by the ever-present influences of friends, family and word-of-mouth. In his words:

> [The] two actors in this psychodrama ... are, and have always been, doctors and patients ... Doctors' notions of what constitutes 'genuine'

6 It is not impossible to imagine, however, an alternate historical or contemporary scenario in which the parameters of respectability were different, and therefore a different mode of illness was 'aped'. Presumably, Shorter would contend that his theory would still hold true in this circumstance, if he were to admit the usefulness of conceiving such a universe.

> organicity may alter, perhaps as a result of increased scientific knowledge or new cultural preconceptions. Although patients' notions of disease tend to follow doctors' ideas … patients may also change their notions of the legitimacy of symptoms that have little to do with medicine.
>
> (Shorter, 1993, pp. x–xi)

To give this idea a little more flesh, let us see how it operates through one of Shorter's examples, reflex theory, which was influential in the second half of the nineteenth century.

In its most basic formulation, this was the idea that any organ in the body could, by means of a 'reflex arc' transmitted through the nervous system of the spine, affect at a distance some other organ or bodily function. In particular, the uterus was seen as a troublesome piece of anatomy (when is it not?), and was the site of growing medical meddling with female reproductive organs. It was thought that, as every internal item was connected dynamically with every other, and since the uterus was believed to be among the most influential of all parts of the female body, it made sense that in some form or other it would be sending nefarious signals to all the things it could reach.

Targeting the uterus as the source of disparate symptoms was not the only method of applying this theory to treatment. Connections between distant body parts were constantly being drawn and redrawn, and remedies included pulling on the tongue in order to galvanise the heart, 'propping up' organs (through surgery) that were said to have fallen out of place and thus caused instability in the nervous system and reflexively generated hysteria, treating breasts to cure a painful womb, and cauterising nasal mucosa to influence 'everything imaginable'.

The immediate result of this theoretical backdrop, according to Shorter, was that patients, mainly women, became fixated on certain areas of the body which are in fact impossible to experience specifically, such as the uterus.[7] Thus, what was vague pain, tiredness or otherwise dissipated and ambiguous distress became funnelled through this analysis into a coherent and centred dysfunction. Though reflex theory is complicated and multifaceted, Shorter demonstrates quite succinctly how a combination of factors and pressures collide under one banner to provide a complete and convenient explanation of disease, which in turn affects treatment and presentation:

> For patients it provided a mooring of certainty in the face of the body's bewildering signals: it was just those pesky pelvic reflexes again. For doctors reflexes provided a general explanation of how disease in one part of the body affected the other parts: nervous signals from any other

7 That is to say, you can certainly experience pain coming from the vicinity, but it is not an organ which you can identify experientially from others around it in the way you could, say, with the lungs or heart.

> irritated organ could travel up and down the spinal cord to any other target organ in the body. In women, the uterus and ovaries were thought the organs most susceptible to irritation, thus the organs that drove forward disease processes elsewhere. But reflexes could also spread to the brain, offering explanations of nervous and psychiatric symptoms in men and women generally, but particularly in women because of the permanent state of irritability of the female pelvis.
>
> (Shorter, 1993, p. 45)

The exact nature of the mechanism whereby culture engenders symptoms, with its changeable weighting over time between doctors, science, other patients and popular media, is difficult to pin down, and I will return to this topic later.

The doctor–patient relationship

From historical continuity and the symptom pool, we move now to what I consider the third important strand of Shorter's thinking, the doctor–patient relationship and the loss of medical authority. He has stated that 'the history of psychosomatic illness is one of ever-changing steps in a *pas de deux* between doctor and patient' and his analysis of the evolving nature of this dance provides some insight into the occasionally antagonistic and counterproductive dynamic that can be witnessed between modern-day sufferers of contested diseases and their various physicians.

Historically, Shorter (1986) identifies and delineates three loose but clear phases in the development of the doctor–patient relationship. The first, *traditional*, refers to the age before the rise of the doctor as a cultural symbol of trust and healing. Roughly speaking, this means pre-1850, and can be defined by a distrustful and dismissive attitude among patients, who for the most part view medicine (accurately) as failing to provide much in the way of diagnostic accuracy or therapeutic efficacy. Following this we entered a period termed by Shorter as *modern*, wherein the doctor became a powerful, respected figure, able to diagnose and explain but in many cases still without the ability to cure with consistency. After the Second World War and just as we entered the age of miraculous medicine, he believes we transitioned to a *postmodern* doctor–patient relationship. This represents a return to a period of cynicism about mainstream medicine, characterised by doctor-shopping, an enormous boom in alternative therapies, increased litigious agitation, the growth of patient communication and networks, the proliferation of new, non-medically sanctioned explanations for illness and the expansion, entrenchment and reduced treatability of psychosomatic conditions. To draw the distinction sharply, until the 1960s, 'near veneration of the doctor was the rule, the demigod in white whose patients would willingly sacrifice their ovaries to suit his theories', whereas following this point 'mistrust of the doctor and refusal to accept his or her reassurance' became the defining feature of doctor–patient interactions in relation to somatisation (Shorter, 1986, p. 299).

What is of relevance to our discussion here is the thesis that Shorter advances regarding the complex relationship between psychogenic conditions, trust in doctors, placebos and the general therapeutic environment of the contemporary world. His basic idea is that over the time-span of the *modern* period, a number of psychogenic complaints, which are the central loci of his historical focus, began in many cases to be treated quite effectively. This is due to a combination of informal psychotherapy within the consultation itself, conducted over a lengthy period of time and incorporated many elements, and a wide range of placebo therapies. Mostly harmless, these suggested cures were often entered into wholeheartedly by patients not only hoping to get better but fully believing that they would do.[8] This is the key, according to Shorter, for understanding why in some cases they did indeed improve: because they felt listened to and respected by a professional, who in turn possessed significant authority and standing, and who was able to explicate their symptoms in cogent, scientific terms (be it spinal irritation, reflex theory, neurasthenia or whatever) which in turn came hand in hand with a treatment programme. By some intuitive though mysterious internal mechanism, this benevolent network of suggestion was able to save a great deal of people a great deal of pain.

Things change, however, when postmodern patients appear. A decline of the doctor as a lionised figure is the result of both push- and pull-factors. On one side, doctors became more and more the agents of scientific fields; immunology, biochemistry and pharmacology were placed above patient and family history and the amount of time spent talking and listening to patient declined as the number of diagnostic tests available increased exponentially. In fact, instances of 'bedside' medicine became anachronisms, eventually disappearing altogether, as doctors' spaces became more and more centralised and their time with patients more and more limited. Medical schools became explicitly biomedical, and student doctors were given 'a picture of disease that ignores the mind'.

On the other side of these trends are developments among patients themselves in the second half of the 20th century. The archetypical patient here is an individualist consumer, who has done their own research, has self-diagnosed, is sure of what they want and is unwilling to accept anything different from their medical practitioner, who finds themselves transformed into a gateway to prescriptions and little else.[9] This is nothing if not a caricature, but it aptly captures medicine's prejudices and fears around this period. Lying

8 The biggest exception to this is the large number of unnecessary surgeries that were performed.

9 This transition in the meaning of the 'patient' from passive receiver of planned, paternal care to active agent in possession choice happened in the UK and elsewhere from the mid- to late 20th century (Mold, 2010; Mold, 2015).

under the surface is a sense that something had gone awry with both the way doctors talks to their patients and the way that patients have come to view their doctors. Shorter certainly takes this stance, and argues that it has had direct ramifications for the way in which psychosomatic conditions are treated (or, as the case may be, not treated).

What these changes have meant is that big chunks of the positive suggestive matrix established in the modern period were eroded, and replaced by systems of care both less effective and more harmful. The biggest aspect of this is pharmacology:

> The problem today is not that patient's don't believe in their doctors' scientific qualities. They do: but that scientific status centres almost exclusively on drugs. The torrent of effective drugs since the 1940s has given medicine a gleaming, high-tech allure. Patients of today go to the doctor because they must go through him to get the drugs that are truly powerful.
>
> (Shorter, 1986, p. 92)

There is a further element to this. Yes, in the place of spa treatments, patients grew to expect specific, targeted drug treatments that mirror approaches to organic disease. But what is also different is the necessary uncertainty that accompanies such therapy. Trial and error tactics with different medications do little to instil the requisite faith in patients that what they are taking will be effective, perhaps summed up by that familiar and formulaic sentence 'we will try you on X, and, if that doesn't work then we'll give you a course of Y'.[10] Without faith, however naïve, the placebo effect ceases to operate.

Shorter adds to this the encroachment of the media into terrain once the sole dominion of medicine. Whereas, in the years of the modern period, medical authority would be largely accepted in areas pertaining to medicine, now we witness a situation where alternate sources of information, sensationalism and epistemic structures more favourable to patient prejudices jostle for space alongside scientific opinion. As Shorter puts it:

> … what is different … is that the authority of the mass media has started to take precedence over what was once called medical authority. The dominant medical paradigms of our own time fall unheeded in the babble of media interviews of physician-enthusiasts and wrenching accounts of patients' suffering.
>
> (Shorter, 1993, p. 314)

We are left with a fairly grim view of the situation. Patients who would perhaps have been helped in the past are now at the mercy of their conditions

10 Known by medics as 'empiric therapy'.

thanks to changes in their expectations and an alienating, dehumanising medical experience. Doctors, as willing to assist as ever, have less time and more of the wrong tools to help such individuals. There is a dark irony in Shorter's thought here: it is just at the point when medicine comes true on its promises and begins to provide us with genuinely widespread, effective responses to disease that we turn back to cynicism and mistrust.

But while he has provided a fairly credible account of trends within the doctor–patient relationship, there is still much that is unexplained or underdetermined.

For instance, he places too much emphasis on the effectiveness of historical treatments of psychosomatic illness. Many, many 'cures' were just as unable to make people feel better as modern treatments, and some, such as unneeded surgeries, institutionalisation and lengthy rest cures, had significantly worse side-effects than current drug courses. Though Shorter himself details the worse therapeutic excesses listed above, he is unable to convincingly reconcile this with his idea of a time when doctors were far more trusted and therefore possessing both more power of placebo and, he implies, to some degree, humanity.

His excavation of the 20th-century patient is also incomplete. There is little space given to the monetisation of medical systems from the 1950s onwards, the increased education levels of the populace, the growth of 'rights' culture, scandals such as that of the thalidomide babies or, indeed, any number of other factors that could be brought into play to help further explain and analyse this breakdown in trust, which Shorter treats as an unambiguously negative development. The basic facts of this breakdown also remain shakily justified: is it really true that modern doctor–patient interactions are characterised by a business-like determination on the part of patients and a cold indifference to pastoral medicine by doctors? I think the likelihood is that this is a highly exaggerated account of what are, nevertheless, real trends.

The criticisms just listed notwithstanding, Shorter does provide one final framework through which to understand contested illnesses, making explicit reference to chronic fatigue and bringing his work closer to the 21st century. It is on to this, the fourth strand, that we now move.

The postmodern patient

After identifying and breaking down the other aspects of his thesis, starting with the historical continuity of psychosomatic disease – the sense that 'people have always possessed some kind of implicit model for analysing their internal sensations, and the quantity and nature of sensation have probably been historically changeless', the notion of a 'symptom pool' and the three-phase gestation of the doctor–patient relationship, Shorter provides us with one further tool with which to dissect the conditions that have made up most of his life's work. He suggests that trends at the end of the last century acted to loosen up traditional social structures and cast individuals adrift on a sea of uncertainty and bodily obsession:

> At the cultural level, these new patterns come from a distinctively 'post-modern' disaffiliation from family life. If the psychosomatic problems of the nineteenth century resulted from an excess of intimacy in the familial psychodrama, those of the late twentieth century have been the result of the opposite phenomenon: a splintering of close personal ties and a lack of intimacy. These changes of the late twentieth century have had the effect of making people more sensitive to bodily signals than ever before and more willing to shift the attribution of their plight from internal demons to external toxins.
>
> (Shorter, 1993, p. 295)

The argument he is making here is that in the second half of the 20th century we, in Western societies, transitioned from a view of the family as a unit worthy of ultimate commitment to a milieu in which the 'desire for self-actualisation' takes precedence. This is symbolically represented by the salience of 'the relationship' (and the willingness to 'shop around' for the best one), at the expense of marriage. Consequences from this shift included a significant decrease in multigenerational cohabitation to the point of near-extinction and a marked increase in people either living alone or with just one partner.[11]

Shorter intimately connects this 'decline' in the traditional family unit with two processes, each of which contribute to an increase in psychosomatic behaviour and fixed illness belief. The first of these is the removal of the checks and balances that others in close proximity provide, something he terms 'feedback loops', an appellation I will avoid as it might cause confusion with my later discussion of Hacking's feedback loops, which are different. What Shorter means by these checks and balances are the normal social dynamics that regulate and reassure us about our health, most often provided by others in our immediate environment. When you remove the partner and the grandparent who would ordinarily serve as a sounding board for health worries and complaints, an individual is left to come to a conclusion by themselves, or via the internet. Therein lies the danger, says Shorter, for in this individualised, unregulated space, obsessive behaviour related to bodily signals develops, not helped by a reliance on mass media or patient groups for further information. Where once there would have been concern but rebuttal, there is now exaggeration and scaremongering.

The second process that Shorter identifies is loneliness. People are now single for longer than before, spend more time living on their own and the elderly in particular are more likely to be socially isolated. This loneliness can breed a discontent that feeds directly into the worries presented above, that of an individual left to appraise their own physical state without the appropriate

11 Though interestingly, this trend has reversed somewhat in the last decade largely due to economic pressures on housing.

tools to do so, compounded by the fact that unhappiness and somatisation have so often gone hand in hand.

Discussion

His work is, of course, already out of date. The growth of the internet has had a large impact on healthcare. The way patients communicate, the sources from which they gather and disseminate information, the very language in which they structure their experiences have all become both more universal (and thus homogeneous) and more rapid. It is difficult to gauge accurately the ways in which a truly connected world has changed the dynamics of diseases such as those under consideration here.[12]

However, Shorter provides us with much more than an antiquated theory. The historical aspect of his work and the ways in which he brings to bear many different factors upon his analysis do provide an answer to the question he sets out to respond to, namely why is it that psychosomatic conditions seem so fluid in their presentation over time and what is it about our current age that would appear so conducive to their proliferation as notoriously difficult, often untreatable entities?[13] In fact, most of his ideas can be applied to modern case studies with a little extension here and there but no real issue. He has provided us with a sophisticated template for understanding certain conditions, one which retains relevance as we move through the first quarter of the 21st century.

At the beginning of this section, I borrowed Hacking's words and described Shorter as a 'highly critical' theorist. He is precisely that. I am not in the least bit surprised that his work has angered patients of one stripe or another. His tone can be sneering and condescending and he oscillates between high scholarship and polemic. What is of more concern, however, is his lack of interest in getting underneath the skin of patients and asking why they behave in the ways that they do, especially in relation to rejecting psychological causes. He recognises the problem, and forensically tracks the various ways that this pattern plays out in the 20th century: the refusal of psychiatric help, the demands for medication, the way that a fixed belief in organicity repeats itself over and over in myriad circumstances. What he fails to do is to provide an adequate framework for understanding this process, beyond basic notions of personal responsibility and stigma. The effect of this theoretical sloppiness, especially in light of the thorough approach he takes to other aspects of this work, is to reinforce the notion that these patients are not worthy of the same respect as other sick people, that they are simply being unreasonable, that

12 That being said, the evidence does suggest that in some cases these changes have had positive ramifications for doctor–patient relations (Iverson, Howard and Penney, 2008; Tan and Gonnawardene, 2017).

13 Note: *an* answer, not *the* answer.

they are overly pliable pawns of their own imaginations and a misguided if solicitous media and communication environment.

A better grasp on the metaphysical conceptions of the patient – how do they see themselves and their condition? – what causes them to, apparently so consistently and without thought, latch on to biological explanations and reject holistic approaches? – would allow a more detailed and nuanced attempt at uncovering the exact mechanism of cultural suggestion that Shorter hangs many of his ideas on. Indeed, the experience of contested disease teaches us that while patients' relationships with medical authority have changed, their clamour for the legitimacy it brings has not lessened. In fact, it is not so much that patients have lost faith in doctors or in medical science, it is that their conditions fall outside of the parameters of biomedicine. If there was a true and absolute loss of medical authority, then the alternate aetiological models proposed would not latch on so enthusiastically to biochemical explanations. The breakdown in trust that is often seen between doctors and patients in this situation is of a more convoluted manner than simply a case of behavioural changes on the patient side and a growing indifference to holistic care on the other; both groups still operate more or less within the same framework, and when conditions emerge that do not fit, the urge of patients is not towards a rejection of medical authority but towards whatever assimilation they can achieve.

A further unresolved tension in this work is the relationship between the 'symptom pool' and patients' subjective feelings. How exactly do trends in scientific understanding, popular culture and the doctor–patient relationship translate into the everyday experience of a body? Shorter describes these factors as forming a 'climate of suggestion', and suggests that the relative importance of one or other at any given time will vary, but the details he provides of this process deserve scrutiny.

For example, he states that the introduction of the Babinski test and the use of ophthalmic diploscopes strongly discouraged the subconscious production of paralysis and achromatopsia; as these conditions became liable to being 'disproved', the body sought new and more difficult to expose forms of organic mimicry. For this to be true, in the strictest sense, a fairly extraordinary level of medical and scientific literacy would be required from the population at large. Evidence that might suggest otherwise is lacking, and it unreasonable to believe that the proliferation of relatively niche scientific ideas and technology occurs both quickly and with regularity.[14]

14 Although there are issues with using science literacy surveys, they consistently present an image of populations that either misunderstand or are ignorant of fairly basic scientific concepts. A relatively recent survey in America, aiming to discover how much effect a college education had on science literacy, concluded 'It appears that high school education and students' exposure to media and popular culture convey a basic knowledge of science, although it is piecemeal and barely adequate' (Impey et al., 2011).

As well as this, his specific ideas about the role of suggestion and symptomatic transference from doctors can at times be vague. While he is well versed in the history of this, suggesting for example that 'the story of Charcot demonstrates the enormous capacity of doctors to frame and shape symptoms which their patients then experience', he is less clear about how this operates under the modern climate of distrust and rejection of medical authority. Perhaps we should understand, by implication, that Shorter believes that in modern circumstances the role of the doctor to mould and influence a patient's symptoms is much reduced.

Alongside the above we must place his claims about the media and popular culture. Sympathetic or exaggerated coverage of a disease, along with a vague description of symptoms, gives individuals what they have been looking for: a box with a scientific name in which to place their body's haywire attempts to communicate with them. They now have a research object with its own distinctive traits, something to bring with them when they visit their doctor, some loose form of closure. And, if they do not see the original article or TV show, perhaps a friend or family member did. The net for such concepts is cast wide in a media-saturated society. This sounds like a fairly neat explanation, but again the question is the same: what exactly is the mechanism and why is it so apparently effective? Are these individuals such unthinking and alike agents that their digestion of and response to media reports is so simple-minded? As we shall see in the second half of this book, the experience of some patients is far more complex than Shorter's theory allows for.

Showalter

There is a significant amount of overlap between Edward Shorter and Elaine Showalter's work, so this section will be reasonably brief as I only intend to discuss elements of her research which challenge or expand his ideas. Like him, she believes that many contentious conditions that populate the modern medical exist on a historical continuity with the unhappy women of the Salpêtrière.[15] And, like him, she believes that medical authority has been eroded to the point of dysfunction and that various public institutions contribute to the creation and perpetuation of illness. However, she is not just a medical historian but also a literary critic, and her analysis barely takes a step in any direction without recourse to language and narrative. A point she powerfully and repeatedly makes is that words and stories shepherd us through our experiences, making sense of them while simultaneously *making them make sense* by smoothing rough edges and incongruities into well worn, recognised

15 'Hysteria has not died. It has simply been relabelled for a new era' (Showalter, 1997, p. 4) – an opinion about which Hacking (2002, p. 89) says 'Showalter is ... profoundly right in saying hysteria is not dead'.

archetypes. As she says (Showalter, 1997, p. 99), 'literature spreads hysteria, but it can also help us understand it'.

Her work in this area is more refined than Shorter's, and presents us with a few answers to the questions I posed immediately above. From her approach we can see more clearly how a symptom pool might come to be assembled and disseminated, and what cultural conditions might contribute to what she has, somewhat hyperbolically, termed 'contemporary hysterical epidemics'.

Showalter's hysteria

There are, she claims, three ingredients necessary for a modern incarnation of hysteria to take shape and proliferate. These are: sympathetic and involved physicians and enthusiasts, disaffected and isolated patients, and a surrounding cultural environment that is conductive to spreading and maintaining false illness beliefs. The first step is for a doctor, scientist or some other person in a position of authority to define, name and publicise a new disorder. This acts as a catalyst for patients looking for a diagnostic label and for some explanation as to what they are feeling. 'The most influential doctors', she writes (Showalter, 1997, p. 17), 'are ... theorists who offer a unified field theory of a vague syndrome, providing a clear and coherent explanation for its many confusing symptoms'. As doctors 'recruit' more patients to their diagnosis, so it is that news of the disease is spread through increased press attention. Eventually, through film and television, novels and plays, self-help books and BBQs with your neighbours, the modes of expressing one particular condition or another become familiar – symptoms and stories congeal and solidify, then appear to provide evidence by their very consistency. All of this takes place against a social background which may be more or less disposed to a certain illness at any specific time. According to Showalter, the 1990s in America represented a particularly fertile soil in which for hysteria to grow: technological advances in telecommunications, the birth of the internet, an increasingly pervasive, increasingly confessional mass media – all these intersect with the 'more generalised paranoias, religious revivals, and conspiracy theories that have always characterised American life'.

Although her appraisal is not without mistakes – most glaringly adopting a one-size-fits-all approach to what are quite clearly different phenomena (she conflates the causal origins of chronic fatigue syndrome, satanic ritual abuse, multiple personality syndrome and alien abduction almost unthinkingly, for example) – she does make some genuinely interesting points about how the process of cultural transference of symptoms might occur.[16] What is most

16 A criticism Simon Wessely echoes (Larkin, 1998). I would agree with Perring when he says, in response to Showalter's sensationalism and generalisation, that we should instead follow 'the humdrum option of taking the middle way, going case by case, and being cautious' (Perring, 1997).

innovative about her characterisation of this mechanism is the emphasis she places on literary devices being played out in real life. As she says:

> Above all, hysteria tells a story, and specialists in understanding and interpreting stories know ways to read it. As hysteria has moved from the clinic to the library, from the case study to the novel, from bodies to books, from page to stage and screen, it has developed its own prototypes, archetypes and plots. Many of these motifs are adapted from myth, popular culture, folklore, media reports, and literature.
>
> (Showalter, 1997, p. 6)

What this leads to, she suggests, is a remarkable convergence of both form and content. Individuals begin to experience their symptoms in the same way and talk about it using the same terminology. Interestingly, she also claims that this symmetry extends to developments in the disease; if the condition changes in some form, then the changes experienced are likely to be consistent among patients as they react subconsciously to alterations in their socio-medical environment. As stories of illness are told and retold, they become concurrently more well-known, more similar and, implicitly, more legitimate by their repetition:

> Patients learn about diseases from the media, unconsciously develop the symptoms, and then attract media attention in an endless cycle. The human imagination is not infinite, and we are all bombarded by these plot lines every day. Inevitably, we live out the social stories of our time.
>
> (Showalter, 1997, p. 6)

There is a further aspect to this. It is not simply the case that these templates always develop organically or in a linear fashion. On occasion they appear entirely deliberate, created and disseminated by professionals, self-help authors, horoscope writers and patient groups themselves. I do not mean that a group of individuals set out to 'create' a disease, but rather that their actions are focused around the things which spread narrative information about a condition, rather than this being an unintended side effect of some other process. And thus it is that disorders become personalised into prototypes, vague enough to apply to a wide number of cases, specific enough to contain heuristic qualities for readers, viewers and listeners, which they use to solidify their conceptual understanding of the disease.

To show how these various ideas of cultural support and prototype development interact in an actual disorder, I will borrow Showalter's convincing example of anorexia from the mid-20th century onwards. The first thing to say is that the surrounding culture in America at that time was broadly sympathetic to the development of such a condition. Aesthetic demands were placed on the female body like never before, with an ideal body type projected across magazine stalls, billboards and cinema screens. Adolescent girls were the vulnerable group most likely to be affected by the obsession with thinness, weight-loss, beauty and exercise. They ate up the popular culture of the 1960s onwards and internalised the messages about beauty and happiness it conveyed. Then, an articulate and well-known authority figure, Hilde Bruch, provided a coherent theoretical framework for anorexia, and through two widely read books popularised her ideas and inserted the basic 'facts' about the illness into the public consciousness. Not only this, but these works outlined what was to become the prototypes of the disease – the quiet, obedient sorts of girls it affected most, the identification of mother–daughter dynamic as especially important, the rejection of natural sexual maturation as a symbolic cause. This information was then replicated in one form or another and circulated through news reports, teen magazines, TV, movies and best-selling novels. After this came celebrity confessions and anorexia autobiographies, as well as a large amount of young adult fiction which tended to vary little in basic plot. Alongside these developments arrived the 'social life' of anorexia, the group counselling sessions, peer-support groups and its assimilation into parts of the feminist movement. It is certainly a compelling picture.[17]

What I think we can take away from this, in conjunction with Shorter's work, is the multitude of obvious and subtle ways that our cultural surroundings structure how we interpret reality. It seems convincing to me that over time an individual might take on board certain pieces of narrative information about a disease and generate from that a series of subconscious expectations and ways of ordering experience that accords with what they have seen, heard or read. This is, I suppose, especially true if the condition is widely known and well publicised.

Another point which Showalter makes that should be considered is the role of fear in gestating hysteria. It is an underlying symbolic theme which runs through her work: where there is an outside force that creates unrest, there are people being made ill by it or understanding their disquiet in opposition to it. As Hacking states:

> Showalter demonstrates how our recent hysterias have one thing in common, a tormented fear of some evil other, from outer space, or from the depths of the soul, or from federal agents, or from the vicious patriarch, or from poisonous gas cocktails in the desert.
>
> (Hacking, 2002, p. 89)

The conditions that concern us in this book do not appear to conform neatly to Showalter's descriptions, however. Conspiracy or outright paranoia for the

17 Though quite clearly not the full picture: who were the anorexics that must have existed in order for Bruch to write about them? How exactly can hearing about other anorexics on the radio *make* you one yourself? These are the sorts of questions that Hacking addresses in detail, so I will leave them for later in the chapter.

most part represents a fringe interest within the patient community, and what we will see in the final part of this book is that for many patients, their first encounter with fibromyalgia or some other contested illness was not through a book or a TV show or some other media, but rather came via a reluctant doctor after months or years of diagnostic uncertainty. Even then, the information they were offered – nebulous and vague aetiologies, inconsistently effective treatment plans – was hardly enough to construct an elaborate and consistent narrative identity. So the question here then is one of degree: in less well-known, less publicised cases, is there less of a prototypical tendency? Showalter would argue that the immense intertextuality of experience in contemporary society means that, whether we realise it or not, there are always narratives to act out or react against. She would also make the point that with conditions like chronic fatigue syndrome and fibromyalgia knowledge *is* widely disseminated, not just through traditional channels but also through patient organisations, regardless of what individual patients might claim.

Showalter makes one further point which I will quickly address. Writing in 1997, she makes explicit links between the surrounding political culture and the rate at which new conditions appear, expand in patient numbers and plays out. She claims that at the end of the 20th century a climate of political paranoia, anti-establishment feeling, millennialism and developments within the feminist movement (pejoratively labelled 'victim feminism') contributed decisively to the growth in numbers of people either being diagnosed or self-diagnosing themselves with new conditions (Showalter, 1997). To these trends I think we can add the continued rise in scale and power of patient groups, the increasing privileging of experiential knowledge and the way in which group identity (whether that is of the immutable or self-defined type) has become of the locus of so much politicised heat and activity (Kaminer, 2000).

There are several questions that need to be asked when thinking about what ingredients we find in contemporary society that might create an environment conducive to the sort of processes Showalter and Shorter describe. Where does medical authority stand now? To what extent does an individual privilege their own ability to generate knowledge about themselves over what others, professional and otherwise, tell them? What narratives are available, which are chosen and why? Through which mediums do patients receive these narratives? Are there patterns? The individual thinker who has done more than any other to bring these questions into focus and provide a theoretical framework for understanding them is Ian Hacking. The final section of this chapter will be devoted to him.

Hacking

A minor motif in Saul Bellow's *Humboldt's Gift* is the protagonist Charlie Citrine's internal reflections on a beaver colony he visits while camping with his children. Next to the lake where the animals live, the Park Service put up a series of billboards which described and categorised the habits, activities and various natural cycles of the beavers. What strikes Citrine as profound is that 'the beavers didn't know a damn thing about this. They just went on chewing and swimming and being beavers' (Bellow, 1975, p. 286). This, he supposes, is the exact opposite of what happens when order is given to people: 'we human beavers are all shook up by descriptions of ourselves. It affects us to hear what we hear. From Kinsey or Masters or Eriksen. We read about identity crisis, alienation, etcetera, and it all affects us' (ibid.).

In other words, the study and theorising about a society alters those within it. When we are grouped or organised according to some principle or other, we react to that grouping: we are happy or sad to see ourselves or be in seen in this or that way, we *change*. Citrine completes this observation by wishing that we could be more like the beavers, indifferent to whatever name or description is given to us.[18]

In a less prosaic way, Ian Hacking concerned himself with this 'beaver problem' for the best part of twenty years. What he set about trying to understand is the way in which classifying individuals acts upon those individuals, changes them as objects of knowledge and thus leads to a further change in classification as part of an ongoing process. This topic, detailed in a series of books and papers, has been termed his 'Making Up People' project. As he says (Hacking, 1996, p. 351), 'it is about how a causal understanding, if known by those who are understood, can change their character, can change the kind of people they are that can lead to a change in the causal understanding itself'.

Roughly speaking, Hacking does not just want to know how it is that categories affect those within them or future categories. He would also like to know how we can ourselves make use of this mechanism, and how it might influence the appearance or disappearance of what he has termed 'transient mental illnesses' – those which seem to arise at a specific place and time and then for some reason fade away from public and medical consciousness. Furthermore, he wants to draw connections between questions of memory, questions of the self and questions of category; in other words, how is it that categorising objects of knowledge fundamentally alters the way individuals not only structure their experiences but also the way they remember their lives and thus the very person that they believe themselves to be?

A multitude of kinds

One of the philosophical traditions in which Hacking situates his work is nominalism, or the naming of things. He argues that alongside natural

18 Citrine's position in the novel is actually slightly more complicated than this, especially as it refers to residents of Chicago and German systems of classification (see Heidsieck, 2007).

kinds – that is, names for groupings that occur in the *real world* – we can place human kinds, which are categories that emerge from the social sciences. In his later work, Hacking dropped the 'human' and replaced it with 'interactive' and likewise refrained from talking of 'natural' kinds in favour of 'indifferent' ones, so I will use this terminology from here on in.

Without wanting to dredge through centuries of philosophy on the topic of natural kinds, it is enough to briefly describe the sort of object of knowledge that Hacking has in mind when he talks of 'indifferent' ones.[19] What he means when he discusses such things are sets that exist (or indeed, simply *may* exist) in nature and which we have sought organised, scientific knowledge about. Some examples might be canonical, like the chemical elements, some fashionable (in the 1990s, when Hacking was writing), like quarks and some simply mundane, like a certain type of corn or particular species of tree. Hacking's realism is fairly broad, but this is not what is interesting. What matters to us here is not whether these objects exist or correspond to some actual reality, but that they are examined, grouped and studied yet remain unchanged by that process.

Interactive kinds are, on the other hand, types of people that are conceptualised and ordered according to some agenda or other.[20] Where indifferent kinds are the preserve of physics, chemistry, biology and all their innumerate subsidiaries, interactive kinds begin life in the 'marginal, insecure, but immensely powerful' social sciences. Hacking outlines them as follows:

> By [interactive] kinds I mean kinds about which we would like to have systematic, general, and accurate knowledge; classifications that could be used to formulate general truths about people; generalisations sufficiently strong that they seem like laws about people, their actions, or their sentiments. We want laws precise enough to predict what individuals will do, or how they will respond to attempts to help them or to modify their behaviour.
>
> (Hacking, 1996, p. 352)

Some examples of this would include women refugees, children with autism, people who commit suicide, alcoholics, multiple personality disorder sufferers and communists. Hacking sketches out four criteria in order to show what might qualify as a human kind. Firstly, he is thinking of kinds that are relevant to some people, that apply to some portion of the population. Secondly, these kinds must in the first instance organise individuals, their actions, their

19 For a good discussion of natural kinds, see Dupré (1995); for Hacking on natural kinds, see Hacking (1991).

20 'Agenda' in this context does not, so to speak, have an agenda. I mean it merely to indicate that there must be *some* motivation present, nefarious or benevolent, in order to create a category of people.

habits and behaviour. Thirdly, they should be kinds which are studied in the human and social sciences, groupings about which it has been deemed interesting or important to gain knowledge. Finally, Hacking adds clarity by saying that 'kinds of people are paramount'. What he means by this is that only when the study of people transforms into our *idea* of that sort of person does it become a human kind. If I research a certain set of individuals but that research does not produce any typological knowledge about their behaviour, their experiences, the causal links between their past and present surroundings and the way they 'appear' in the world, then I have not contributed to making a human kind.

As is immediately obvious, the variety of interactive kinds present in a particular society at any one time is immense.[21] Some are too mundane to waste much thought over, such as perhaps (though maybe not historically) 'left-handed people', and, though qualifying as interactive kinds, the truths produced by our knowing about them will indeed be *so* general that there seems little point in pursuing them without qualification or some specificity. There does exist however, apart from these instances, an enormous number of what we might term *useful* interactive kinds. These are groupings on which we might want and hope to have an effect upon through understanding the nature of the effect of categorisation and the many tributaries which contribute to its general flow. They tend to be narrow enough to produce semi-solid truths about which we can talk with a degree of certainty not granted to those broader, more ambiguous groupings. It is these sets that Hacking is most interested in. They form the interactive kinds that he uses as examples and the groupings he thinks the most worthy of analysis.

The way in which he has separated these interactive kinds from indifferent kinds is contested. At its most fundamental, he distinguishes them by saying that the act of categorising an indifferent kind does not alter it, whereas placing an external theoretical structure upon an interactive kind does. As he states:

> Inanimate things are, by definition, not aware of themselves … Take the extremes, women refugees and quarks. A woman refugee may learn that she is a type of person and act accordingly. Quarks do not learn they are a certain type of entity and act accordingly … The idea of quarks does not interact with quarks. Quarks are not aware that they are quarks and are not altered simply by being classified as quarks. There are plenty of questions about this distinction, but it is basic.
>
> (Hacking, 1999, p. 32)

21 Though Hacking is at pains to note that his ideas apply (accurately) only to his society ('My culture is my culture and none other'; Hacking, 1996, p. 351) and require an infrastructure of study ('All classifications that stick exist only within practices and institutions'; Hacking, 2004, p. 285).

I take this to mean that self-consciousness is one of the key distinctions between the two sorts of kinds that are being described: 'naming' something clearly has a different effect on that thing depending on whether or not it is able to absorb, reject or otherwise react to its 'naming'.

A second way in which interactive kinds are said to be removed from indifferent ones is their dynamic nature. Not only does placing a person within a certain grouping, about which we suppose we have knowledge, change them, it also leads to an alteration of the grouping itself, because its subject entities have now shifted and become something else. This means that when we create an interactive kind what we have produced is a moving target. Dynamic nominalism, as this is known, is 'the belief that systems for classifying people created by society may affect what people do, which may in turn affect our knowledge of them' (Schmaus, 1992, p. 169).

Aware that none of his rules will apply in all circumstances, Hacking splits up interactive kinds into various types, producing sub-theories for each. For example, he recognises that in some cases the individual does not *themselves* need to be aware of a classification which applies to them. It is enough in these instances for the surrounding social environment of the person to be influenced. An example he uses to illustrate this – a type of interactive kind he terms inaccessible – is strongly autistic children. These types of people are 'human beings who cannot understand' and for whom there 'cannot be self-conscious feedback'. However, what does possess self-consciousness is the 'larger human unit' that the autistic child is situated in, and this can change depending on what knowledge is produced about the individual in the centre. Thus, as causal understandings change over time (from feeble-mindedness to childhood schizophrenia to refrigerator mothers to theories of mind, etc.), the immediate social and institutional environment of the person so-described is altered. Individuals may also fall in and out of classification depending on such alterations.

This type of kind is important because it appears to challenge Hacking's foundational distinction of self-consciousness, but he does not take it to be a critical flaw. Rather, by expanding the unit of classification beyond the individual to their immediate social surroundings, he argues he is purporting a broader self-consciousness and making the same point – organising a set of qualities and attributing them to a group of people changes both the people and the group – about autistic children as about any other interactive kind.

Inaccessible kinds are not the only subdivisions of interactive kinds that Hacking outlines. He also includes administrative, second-order, biologised and self-ascriptive kinds in his analysis.[22] It is the last two of these which I think are of most relevance here, and which I would like to discuss.

22 Briefly, the first two kinds not discussed at length are as follows (bear in mind there is significant overlap between them and the others). Administrative: kinds created by the categorisation of people into administrative entities, i.e. the interaction between census criteria and those who fall within census criteria ('Hispanic'

'Biologised' kinds represent for Hacking one of the most important and powerful trends in scientific and social thought at the end of the 20th century: the move towards finding genetic or neurological explanations for behaviour that was previously explained as social or environmental.[23] What we find with biologised kinds is that they have a tendency to possess an amorality or absolve responsibility for certain actions. A kind of people whose causal matrixes are formed at birth are different from a kind who *decide* to do something, based on some other reason and influenced by other factors.

This can lead to an interesting tension between competing frameworks which both claim to explain the same phenomena. Hacking gives the example of alcoholism, where one framework – Alcoholics Anonymous – produces knowledge about alcoholics which is explicitly moralistic, and thus creates a different kind of person than that produced by a biologised explanation which 'blames' genetic inclination towards addiction, or changed neural pathways following an initial exposure. Which kind becomes dominant depends on the social context in which the kind is expressed: which kind fits in most with people's preconceived, existing ideas of that sort of behaviour? Who speaks from the position of most authority when defining the kind? Which kind aligns most with other trends present? Which kind of kind do people most want to be? In many cases there is no 'winner' so to speak, and different kinds have precedence in different situations.

When Hacking talks about 'self-ascriptive' kinds, what he is referring to is an inversion of the traditional way in which interactive kinds operate and have operated. Roughly speaking, pre-1950 (according to Hacking), the two axes of the social sciences – a positivist aping of natural science methods and interpretations of causation, and the bureaucratic-statistical mass collection of data – combined to loosely create between them the knowledge and the known. Speaking from the point of view of experts, be it census collectors, sociologists, psychiatrists or whomever, '"we" know about "them"'. That is to say, there is a one-directional model of knowledge production. The known-about remain passive and do not contribute to the creation of knowledge about themselves, except in a subconscious manner. What we have seen since then, says Hacking, is the explosion of a different sort of process, whereby the

is given as a good example). Second-order: these are kinds derived from a primary concept, the most prominent being normality. Once you have an established 'norm' in relation to whatever it may be, deviations from this produce 'abnormal' kinds, the interactive axis being between individuals perceptions of themselves and their perception of what it is to be 'normal', alongside an evaluative element that judges how much this matters, whether it is positive, etc.

23 Hacking does point out that this is in some sense a rerun of previous research programmes from before the Second World War and in the 19th century, but what is different here is both the sophistication of the tools and the lack of an specific ideological driver beyond reductionism and moral exculpation for all within the kind (rather than, say, a specific race).

'known may overpower the knowers'. This inversion is even more marked now than when Hacking was writing, with identity narratives prevalent across the western world which prioritise and valorise self-identification, a trend perhaps taken to its most absurd conclusion (thus far) in the case of Rachel Dolezal.

Self-ascription in this context is where the objects of knowledge themselves lay claim to the epistemic process, and begin opting in or out of a category, generating and disseminating new information and generally challenging the moral and semantic scaffolding of the grouping. What is different about these 'self-ascriptive' kinds is that the motivation behind 'reclaiming' or 'reframing' the interactive kind is almost universally attempted in order to benefit those under description. Classifications can affect the way we evaluate our personal worth, and frequently they represent straightforwardly moral distinctions. Because of this, it can be greatly in the interest of an individual to try and deliberately shift the grouping they believe they are a part of towards something that allows them and others like them more self-respect and emotional contentment, as well as better treatment by others and by institutions whose actions in relation to them are directly organised on the basis of their category.

The canonical example in this respect is homosexuality, which during the last hundred years or so has gone in the West from a top-down (pejorative) medical description of behaviour to a contested psychiatric diagnosis, to a 'lifestyle choice', to a relatively accepted, in some places, way of biologically *being*, with many stops and reversals in between. What is key to this process is the way in which the 'known', homosexuals, fought with the 'knowers' over the category that came to a greater or less extent to define them, and to some degree gained control of the agenda.

These two types of interactive kind often intersect. This is because, generally speaking, self-ascribing kinds push towards biologising as a way of creating a more positive, less stigmatised kind to belong to. This process occurs in virtually any kind in which those involved both feel they are held responsible for their (negative) actions by some portion of society and that their moral condition could be alleviated by pursuing a biological explanation.

To bring this discussion full circle, it is the presence of a moral dimension which is the final substantive wedge between indifferent and interactive kinds. Interactive kinds are imbued with intrinsic normative qualities in a way that indifferent kinds are not. To put it starkly, as Hacking (1996, p. 366) does, 'caked mud and polarized electrons may be good or bad depending on what you want to do with them, but child abuse is bad and multiple personality is a disorder to be healed'.

Hacking is aware that his approach does not accurately outline all of the various links between institutions and the types of people they describe, or indeed the form that those many variations might take. What lies beneath his theories is a belief in the plurality of interactive kinds but also a conviction that this plurality is trivial. Every interactive kind will be different in some way, both from those around it and those that came before, but like Wittgenstein's famous family resemblances, each will have similarities with some others and the overlapping mesh will grant us enough similarity to speak with relevance about them as a group. It is not just regarding interactive kinds that Hacking is a pluralist, but also about the *looping effect of interactive kinds*, a conceptual innovation which we will now examine.

The looping effect of interactive kinds

As outlined above, the most fundamental differences between indifferent and interactive kinds are the self-consciousness, moral content and dynamism of the latter. The mechanism by which these special features affect the categorisation itself and generate a 'moving target' has been termed 'the looping effect' and is key to understanding how producing new knowledge about people causes them to become different and thus our understanding of them to change in an ongoing process.

Essentially, when a category of people is delineated from society on the whole, and knowledge is created and disseminated, institutionally, instrumentally or in some other manner, the individuals in question react. This reaction appears under many guises and is never exactly the same across different kinds. However, in all cases it creates a type of person who is different from that originally under study, with new causal truths and new typologies. Thus the original category is now no longer isomorphic with the object of study, and so must itself change to catch up, analysing, assimilating or rejecting the new knowledge in the same way that the individuals did in the first place. This unfolding and permanently unfinished relationship is what Hacking calls the 'looping effect'.

His best and most extensive example of this is multiple personality disorder, now called dissociative identity disorder, which he chronicled in *Rewriting the Soul*. In this work he outlined two main processes. Firstly, he showed how memory came to be medicalised as a surrogate, secular soul and how trends in the study of hypnotism, fugue, sleepwalking, hysteria and epilepsy shaped this. Secondly, he demonstrated how similar issues of memory and the self played out in a completely different arena: multiple personality disorder (MPD) in 1980s America.

His account, simplified, goes like this. From the first (modern) diagnosis, a prototype 'multiple' is produced and some knowledge about them is distributed. Then, as more psychiatrists become aware of the diagnostic category, they begin to diagnose more multiples, which in turn attracts further press attention.

At this point, the category itself begins to move, or 'wander'. Where once it was a condition that typically presented in patients as a splitting of personality into one or two 'alters' (that is, alternate personalities), soon patients were appearing with more and more, hundreds even. Being abused as a child is identified as a key causal link to adulthood MPD, and this becomes a well-known 'fact' about the condition. Patients who do not recall being abused are encouraged to search their memory and in some cases false memories are recalled, with all the family-splitting acrimony that inevitably arises from incorrect accusations. Journals are started about the condition, conferences are organised and all the while patient numbers grow and grow. There is a backlash: the False Memory Syndrome Foundation is formed to combat misremembered or entirely untrue allegations of sexual abuse made by patients against family members, while some psychiatrists begin to embark on treatment programmes contrary to orthodoxy.

What we witness here, says Hacking, is the complicated interplay between individuals, institutions and the knowledge that flows from one pole to the other. Narrative similarity in patients becomes regarded as evidence for this or that law-like regularity, which in turn suggests to patients that this is a way of structuring their experience. Morality flickers in the background at all stages, steering decisions made by professionals and those caught up in it all, the families and friends of patients. Those themselves who sit at the centre of the whole thing, the individuals in the group, being told what it is they have by different sources, begin to see themselves as someone new, someone different from before. In doing so, says Hacking (2006), they also *become* something different from before, an original type of person:

> We think of many kinds of people as objects of scientific enquiry [and] we think of these kinds of people as given, as definite classes defined by definite properties. As we get to know more about these properties, we will be able to control, to help, to change, or to emulate them better. But it is not quite like that. They are moving targets because our investigations interact with the targets themselves and change them. And since they are changed, they are not quite the same kind of people as before. The target has moved. That is the looping effect. Sometimes our sciences create kinds of people that in a certain sense did not exist before. That is making up people.

It is this last point which is the most profound that Hacking makes, and which is vital to understanding the whole enterprise. When he speaks of 'making up people', what he is referring to is not just a process whereby people evolve. He is articulating something different: categorising people creates not just a modified version of that group but whole new people, people that didn't and couldn't have existed before.[24] The restructuring of experience which comes with new categories and creates new, distinct selfhoods is the final piece of the puzzle required to understand Hacking's interactive kinds.

24 I mean this in a metaphysical sense: the components of selfhood necessary to view yourself in a certain manner, to understand and, more importantly, *process* new experiences, did not exist previously, and therefore *being* this sort of person was not an option.

It is banal to state that as we gain knowledge about the world we begin to organise our experience of it differently. Understandings of the external world and who we are as people lead us to interpret situations and phenomena in ever unfolding ways. To employ some archetypes, a writer may find that they can no longer enjoy the simple pleasures of watching a sunset without the internal compulsion to translate it into prose, the art lover may become unable to hear of an event without picturing the scene in the manner of a corresponding masterpiece and the economist might find themselves frequently conceptualising events according to pieces of financial theory.[25] These restructurings of experience are constant and multifarious: the first time I drove on the motorway at night, for example, I was viscerally reminded of racing games I used to play as a child on the PlayStation, that previous embedded experience informing how my mind processed sensory information in the present.

How Hacking makes use of this idea is far more significant however. He says that new categories of people, new interactive kinds, give individuals unanticipated and unpredictable tools with which to understand their pasts. So it is that as we witness, for example the expansion of categorical, causal knowledge of child abuse, people begin more and more to view themselves as abused and to slot into *that* kind. They restructure their past experiences in light of current knowledge, and so what was viewed as one thing becomes another. This is salient because for Hacking memory is key in modern Western societies to understanding the construction of self.[26] Memory makes us who we are, and if our memory changes, then we become a new type of person.

This process is described as follows:

> New meanings change the past. It is reinterpreted, yes, but more than that, it is reorganised, repopulated. It becomes filled with new actions, new intentions, new events that caused us to be as we are. I have to discuss not only making up people but making up ourselves by reworking our memories.
>
> (Hacking, 2002, p. 6)

More specifically, regarding MPD, Hacking states that:

> A certain picture of origins is imported to disturbed and unhappy people, who then use it to reorder or reorganise their conception of their past. It

25 A character in the Jean Thompson short story 'Applause, Applause' puts it like this: '… this heightened self-awareness was a sign of strain. As if he couldn't really escape his work or the persona that went with it. The Artist's impressions of a walk in the woods. The Artist's view on viewing. The Artist on Art…One ended, of course, by losing all spontaneity. You saw people as characters, sunsets as an excuse for similes …' (Thompson, 1977, p. 233).

26 I mean construction in the strict sense here, i.e. of composite parts, rather than 'social' construction.

> becomes their past. I am not saying their past is directly created by doctors. I am saying that this picture becomes disseminated as a way of thinking of what it was like to be a child and to grow up. There is no canonical way to think of our own past. In the endless quest for order and structure, we grasp at whatever picture is floating by and put our past into its frame.
>
> (Hacking, 2002, p. 88)

Though I would take issue with the ambiguity of his final sentence, on the basis that some 'pictures' are more convenient for our mental and moral wellbeing than others, I think he makes a vitally important point about categories, memory and self-conception. Only when we appreciate that knowledge production about a set of people can deeply, fundamentally alter the way they are can we see the true power of the looping effect.

This restructuring does not of course only extend backwards. New categories also create new possibilities for understanding experience extending into the future, and more dramatically, for new actions. To use a current example, the proliferation of a certain type of pornography (violent, demeaning to women) since the 1990s and especially following its widespread and inexpensive distribution on the internet has had an effect on the way that many individuals conceptualise 'normal' sexual relations, even if that effect is not total mimicry. Further to this internal reclassification, it has produced prototypical sexual experiences and normalised what were more likely to be in the recent past relatively rare sexual events. In many cases, it is simply that individuals had fewer modes of action from which to choose from previously, and the expansion of the possibilities given to them leads to a pattern of behaviour which is self-reinforcing. Hacking makes this point regarding the dissemination of information about child abuse: not only did it lead people to come to see themselves as abused, it also *gave abusers ideas.*

One thing that I think is worth mentioning is Hacking's desire, with MPD, to describe and analyse an interactive kind that was still in motion. A reason why he did this was to show how types of people that may seem concrete categories are actually in an undulating and messy state of constant redescription, and that this is happening all around, all the time. Though possible contemporary instances of this abound, I think the transgender movement is an almost-too-perfect case of this 'still in motion' kind.

Over the last decade or so, we have witnessed a significant growth in the number of people who identify themselves as being transgender. This has come to be seen as a far wider grouping than its antecedent category, transsexual, with a diverse array of meanings, terminology, medical and commercial infrastructure, not to mention a number of legal *causes célèbres* and backlashes of varying size from doctors, journalists, feminist academics and others. I am confident that what we are seeing here is, in Hacking's sense, a *new* type of person. As Carl Elliott (2000) writes (of transsexuals), 'fifty years ago the suggestion that tens of thousands of people would someday want their genitals surgically altered so that they could change their sex would have been ludicrous. But it has happened.'

In transgender people we have all the outward features of an interactive kind – the conferences, the journals, the patient organisations, the biologising, the jargon, the exponential growth of people self-identifying, social contagion, etc. But we also see this intriguing forwards/backwards realignment of meanings; individuals who come to have possession of knowledge about themselves begin reinterpreting the past and the future, and do so in a way which is novel, which has not happened before. The transgender person of today, fighting back against an irreducible cocktail of biologically and culturally defined gender roles, living their life in a societal and political context in which self-ascribed personal identity has emerged as a pivotal force, seeing themselves as a manifestation of, alongside many other things, the right to choose your own way of seeing gender, is a different kind of person than, say, the boy in the 1980s who liked wearing women's clothes because they made him feel more at peace, was regarded as effeminate and grew up to be a gay man (for a critical account, see Brunskell-Evans and Moore, 2018). They are probably even substantially different from the transsexuals seeking surgery that Elliott was referring to in 2000. These things move fast.

Placed together, Hacking's ideas about interactive kinds, the looping effect and the ongoing construction and reconstruction of self appear an attractive and poetic explanatory framework, but to what degree can his theories actually help us to understand individual cases? Is he right about the primary level of looping? And what insight can his theory lend to contested illness?

Discussion

Hacking has stated that he has been accused of being too ironic in his intellectual stance and that people complain he places too much space between himself and his subject matter.[27] The basic claim is that his style negates taking a stand. I disagree with this assessment. His writing does obscure his position, it is true. Partly this is down to his distaste of social constructivism, to him an overtly moral exercise and one from which he wishes to distance himself.[28] Partly too it is because he writes about topics which are current and which inspire histrionics, another style of expression he wants to avoid.

27 'There's too much irony in my work, there really is … People often ask: so you've given us all the options and you've given us good things and bad things about all of them but what the heck do you think? … In general it is a defect in the way that I proceed that I am often very ironical' (in Hacking, 2009).

28 Although, reading *The Social Construction of What?*, you get the distinct feeling that a large part of his problem with social construction is linguistic: he has a certain definition of 'construction' in mind, that of various materials being gathered together and employed to create something new, where a plan is followed

However, beneath this, there *is* a quiet, but distinct, moral agenda. He is not interested in telling people how to live their lives, or in saying that there is a right way to remember or structure your experiences. He is not arguing in favour of one kind of identity over another. But what he is saying is that people are often unhappy and that they may be being harmed by some of the processes he has outlined. Previously stable or treatable people may come to understand themselves in a way which is not amiable to their recovery. The meanings that guide their lives may have been hijacked by one force or another. By mapping these mechanisms, by understanding the different ways in which these things can occur, I think Hacking is hopeful that in some small way we might be able to gain a measure of purchase on their levers. Especially in light of his work regarding memory, identity and the soul, it is fair to say that in some instances the stakes are very high indeed.

This is why it is particularly worrying to consider that his causal understandings may be even more incomprehensible than the 'complex and shady' description of them he allows. Without some degree of applicability, this theory is unable to gain any traction on individual units of study, or be usefully engaged on subjects outside of his own examples.

This is a problem not just of conceptual messiness, but also of specificity. By adhering to a model of looping which assumes each and every instance of looping will be different in some way, there is a risk that we arrive at a situation where every phenomenon requires in-depth, rigorous and extensive historical research in order to be understood. By the time we are able to do this, to work out the particular manifestation of interaction in any given case, that case is likely to have moved on, the 'target' advancing in new and unpredictable directions.

The question, then, is twofold. Hacking is 'explicitly sceptical about the possibility of generating a substantial and generalizable theory of the looping effect' and 'he appears to think that forms of looping are too varied and always highly dependent on specific sociocultural contexts' (Kuorikoski and Pöyhönen, 2012, p. 194). So does this mean, firstly, that his theory is in fact fairly blunt? And could it be modified, clarified or extended in a way that sharpens it?

Tekin (2014) identifies the complexity and ambiguity present in the causal trajectory of the looping effect as a shortcoming of Hacking's approach. She separates this issue into two problematic elements: the lack of an empirically and philosophically cogent account of the self, which sits at the centre of Hacking's theory but is never satisfactorily articulated, and the failure to properly engage with the manifold complexity of psychopathology.

In addressing the first of these sub-problems, the 'missing self', Tekin argues that by showing the looping effect through large examples, Hacking

according to an agenda, etc., which makes the metaphor as it is used in the humanities look decidedly lazy.

has negated providing us with a cogent explanation of exactly *how* and *why* the looping effect influences subjects, causing them to respond in the way that they do. She points out that although Hacking talks of the person/subject/self/soul interchangeably, his focus is their interactions, not them, and therefore he does not 'delve into *what* it is about that self that is prone to being made up' (Tekin, 2014, p. 232; emphasis in original). In other words, how uniform is the pattern of looping? What factors make a person more or less likely to react in a certain way to their classification? Why are some people presented as pliable and suggestible but others seem more robust? In essence, what motivates changes in self-concepts and behaviour? I think these are all serious questions that Hacking does not address.

In her analysis of the second unexplained aspect of the looping effect, Tekin focuses on psychopathology as a specific case or category, and the varying weight we should give to its different axes – classification, subjective symptoms, knowledge about diagnosis, etc. She is right to point out that the relationship between these factors is not adequately examined by Hacking. Three questions, says Tekin, remain:

- How much of the change in the subject's self-awareness and behaviour is connected to the knowledge they receive about the diagnosis?
- How much of such change is connected to their particular mental disorder?
- How much of the change in their self-concept and behaviour is connected to the clinical treatment they receives upon diagnosis?

In short, she is arguing that in cases of psychopathology, and I would posit other conditions as well, the looping effect is not just mediated by the knowledge received by the patient about their classification, but also by their clinical encounters and the actual course of their illness. There are in essence many different, overlapping loops interacting with one another at the same time, and that Hacking fails to elucidate and situate these other potential influences in detail is a weakness of his approach. I would add one further question, of a more general nature, to Tekin's three:

- How much does the immediate social environment of an individual alter their self-concept?

Hacking has already discussed how the 'larger human unit' that surrounds an autistic child or other inaccessible kind can influence looping, but I think he underestimates the impact that family, social and workplace environments can have on a person's relationship to their category and themselves. Partly this is due to intellectual positioning. Though he acknowledges his debt to both, to me Hacking is clearly further towards Foucault's top-down, institutional study of meanings than Goffman's bottom-up approach. He is instinctively more interested in how large, organising bodies of epistemic production affect individuals under their gaze than how interpersonal relationships with others might produce similar effects. This could just be because he is a philosopher and not a sociologist, and because using Foucauldian methods have a tendency to produce Foucauldian results.[29]

It may be in fact that it is a several step process, where the first arc of looping is indeed directed by institutions and social scientists. But I would posit that after this stage the direction of such loops becomes muddied. Other members of society, not in the group themselves but aware of its classification, may come to have a more important role in generating feedback relationships.

Goffman (1969) wrote about this in *The Insanity of Place*. This work represented a shift in focus from the more institutional, closed-system type analysis of *Asylums* (Goffman, 1961) towards an intimate and probably highly autobiographical account of illness in a family setting (Shalin, 2014). He recognised the immense power of feedback within an immediate social setting and how it might slot in with other factors such as diagnosis and institutionalisation. Hacking does, on the face of it, acknowledge the potential relevance of such an intersection:

> Goffman's idea of looping applies to one rather well-understood phenomenon of face-to-face interaction. Mine, much less well understood, applies to a quite different phenomenon bearing on classification itself. Yet it is very probably that my kind of looping, at the abstract level of discourse, works only because of Goffman's concrete looping effect, at the interpersonal level of face-to-face interaction.
>
> (Hacking, 2004, p. 299)

I would say that this is incorrect, or at least incomplete. What Hacking is arguing is that his looping effect is between the classification and the classified, that this is a dynamic relationship of change, and that this is perhaps sustained by face-to-face interaction. What I would argue is that once the ball is rolling, so to speak, it is often the wider social context of an individual, represented by constant interpersonal and now online encounters, which affects their relationship with their category.[30] *This*, in some cases, causes more change, more 'movement' of the interactive kind, than anything else. Therefore, the broader social environment's reaction to the classification (and indeed the broader social environment's *understanding* of the classification) of

29 'As a research strategy, I have always been much taken by what Michel Foucault named archaeology. I think that there are sometimes fairly sharp mutations in systems of thought and that these redistributions of ideas establish what later seems inevitable, unquestionable, necessary' (Hacking, 2002, p. 4).

30 Or, as Goffman writes, 'the third parties, the patient's daily circles: his service community, his work place, his friendships and particularly his family' (Goffman, 1969, p. 360).

the individual is what has caused the kind to shift and become something new, not their personal interactions with their category. Most crucially, subsequent changes in the institutional categorisation of an individual may well have little effect on the way they are classified socially, and thus may be of limited impact in relation to the dynamism of the interactive kind.

I do not think that it is controversial to emphasise the importance of this level of looping. Individual's identities are constituted and reconstituted continuously on the basis of our interactions with others. We come to think of ourselves as being *this* way and not *that* way only within a social matrix, and it informs the way we interpret present and past events and actions. Sometimes we are even self-aware enough to realise that this process is occurring as it does so. In Doris Lessing's *The Golden Notebook*, for example, the narrator Anna Wolfe is acutely conscious of the impact that being part of one or other grouping can have on social relations. Anna describes an encounter with an old friend after she had joined the Communist party:

> The fact I had become a party member, made me, for her, an embodiment of something she had to have certain attitudes towards. And I responded in kind. At which Michael said: 'Well, what did you expect?' He was speaking in his role of East European exile, to me in my role as 'political innocent'. And I replied in that role, producing all sorts of liberal inanities. Fascinating – the roles we play, the way we play parts.
>
> (Lessing, 2007, p. 153)

It is fairly obvious what Anna (or perhaps Doris) is getting at here, that our categories change not just how we see ourselves but how the whole world sees us, which in turn alters how we view our identity and how we act. And I believe that this line of thought – that the social environment is paramount in looping – has gained particular salience given the events of the decade or so since Hacking stopped writing substantially on this topic. In 1996 he wrote that 'there has been a bizarre proliferation of self-help groups of late. Their core feature has been self-ascription: their rhetoric is that of taking control of themselves' (Hacking, 1996, p. 351).

I would argue that due to a number of factors, most notably the internet's galvanising effect on communication and the influence of individualist, identity-based movements, self-ascription is in many cases now the norm (Franck, 2000). With contested illnesses, disease identities have been continuously fought over and negotiated at the theoretical level, and though they are still a case-study in uncertainty and diagnostic ambiguity, a sufficiently acceptable conceptual framework for several diseases has been established.

Patients in many cases now have little conflict with their institutional category (relatively speaking) because of the variety of meanings that are available and because of the hand they play in shaping those meanings themselves. The greatest source of tension that has evolved is not between classifiers and classified, because to some extent these have become one and the same, but between the classified and everyone else. These 'others', for whom the category means one thing or another (normally, in the eyes of patients, a retrograde and pejorative set of assumptions), are the boundary at which individuals react most to their grouping. It is these relationships and the tensions within them, not to mention their effects, that we will look at in detail in the second half of this book.

Part 2

Contested illness in context

Chapter 5

Fibromyalgia

Introduction

At the beginning of this book, I explained that my aim was to examine contested disease in a philosophical context, or rather, in *its* philosophical context. To do this I have so far talked in general terms, stretching and teasing at the edge of concepts to test their robustness, and have outlined a number of overlapping frameworks that might aide our understanding of the experiences patients have. It is these experiences around which this half of the book is based, the idea being to search for the contours of what might loosely be termed 'our general understanding of disease' or the 'prevailing notions of legitimate illness'.

Focusing on this is important, as it links into all sorts of other epistemic points I wish to make – that the reality of disease for many people is greatly affected not just by 'medical' knowledge (in so far as it is possible to bracket this), but by the underlying metaphysical beliefs of the population at large and more specifically the population around the diseased person: their family, friends, work colleagues and indeed to a great degree themselves. In the same way that phenomenological work on illness has exposed the various physical aspects of our environment that we take for granted, I would like to chip away at our understanding of disease and uncover the presumptions, the intuitions, the expectations that shape our view of an ill person in our vicinity or in the mirror.[1]

In this half of the book I will focus on one contested disease in particular: fibromyalgia, an outline of which I shall now provide.

Characteristics

Fibromyalgia is characterised by widespread musculoskeletal pain across the body, fatigue, cognitive issues and other symptoms. Patients are often

1 Phenomenology is not alone in this achievement – many years of disabilities rights activism have likewise highlighted the 'able-bodiedness' of our designed environments.

comorbid with a range of psychological conditions such as depression and anxiety as well as other contested illnesses like chronic fatigue syndrome and irritable bowel syndrome. Fibromyalgia's aetiology is a site of conflict and no one model exists which can adequately map the disease. Likewise, the diagnostic tools used to demarcate the condition are also called into question.

As with many of the ailments it is often placed alongside, fibromyalgia has a troubled and oblique genealogy (for a more exhaustive history of the concept, see Inanici and Yunus, 2004). To those prone to scouring history, confirmation bias in hand, examples of chronic pain, muscular discomfort and fatigue stretch from the Bible to Shakespeare. These are of less interest to us, however, than the modern, explicitly diagnostic attempts to classify what remains an uncertain symptom constellation.

Although discussion of rheumatism, muscle sensitivity and tenderness can be found among physicians throughout the 19th century, the first reference to 'fibrositis' seems to appear in 1904, as used by Sir William Gowers. He hypothesised that an unknown process which inflamed the fibres of the lumbar muscles was the cause of backache (Malleson, 2002). A contemporary physician of his named Ralph Stockman used the term more broadly to describe patients with symptoms that align quite isomorphically with modern presentation (stiffness and aching, muscular fatigue, general pain), and throughout the 20th century these vague complaints were variously swallowed by a number of diffuse classificatory frameworks, patients being assigned different labels and finding themselves under the care of various specialisms.[2]

It was not until the 1970s that 'fibrositis' again caught the sustained attention of rheumatologists and began to stimulate clinical interest, leading directly to the dissemination of the diagnostic criteria that brought 'fibromyalgia' into existence (Goldenberg, 2009, pp. 12–13). This began with Smythe (1972), who sketched an outline of the condition that included much of what we now take to be of central importance: generalised muscle pain, fatigue, disrupted and low-quality sleep, aggravation through exertion, potential underlying emotional distress and multiple tender points. Further work was completed which emphasised the role that disturbed and unusual sleep patterns played in the aggravation of symptoms, and by 1983 key researchers were calling upon the field of rheumatology to produce reliable diagnostic criteria which could be used to accurately classify the disease now known as 'fibromyalgia' (Hench 1976; Moldofsky et al., 1978; Yunus, 1983). This was provided in 1990 by the American College of Rheumatology (ACR), who placed the presence of eleven (or more) out of eighteen possible 'tender points' at the centre of distinguishing between fibromyalgia patients and those with other conditions, these providing the 'most discriminating power', alongside widespread pain (Wolfe, Smythe and Yunus, 1990).

2 Myofascial syndrome, neurasthenia, post-infectious fatigue, myasthenic syndrome, myalgic encephalomyelitis, myofasciitis and muscular rheumatism, for example.

Subsequent to this, research interest increased alongside rising patient numbers. It was clear that fibromyalgia patients presented with far more than simply tender points, and that the routine diagnostic test proposed by the 1990 criteria was rarely being used or was being used incorrectly. As a result, fibromyalgia became regarded as a 'dustbin diagnosis' or diagnosis of exclusion, a label given to patients when all other diagnostic options had been exhausted.

Though the ACR criteria stimulated plenty of research, along genetic, epidemiological, haematological and more general pathophysiological lines, this failed to translate into effective clinical practice, where diagnosis remained uncertain, treatment inconsistent and outcomes poor. In light of these problems, the ACR revised their criteria in 2010, introducing the use of widespread pain index (WPI) and symptom severity scale (SS) scores alongside a requirement that symptoms be present for at least three months or more and the presence of no other disorders which might better explain the symptoms (Wolfe et al., 2010).

Current clinical debates

Fibromyalgia, or fibromyalgia syndrome as it is often referred, is characterised by widely distributed, chronic musculoskeletal pain, as well as elements of fatigue, joint stiffness, cognitive difficulty, sleep disturbances, headaches, bowel problems and other symptoms (this section is drawn largely from: Chinn, Caldwell and Gritsenko, 2016; Clauw, 2014; Bellato et al., 2012). The pain is often variable and patients report that the intensity of their symptoms appears to be related to stress and physical exercise. Common patient conceptualisations of their symptoms include 'fibrofog', which is the inability to remember pieces of information, the clouding of an otherwise functional mind, and 'flare ups' which refer to a particularly bad symptomatic reaction to something, such as stress, physical overexertion or changes in the weather.[3]

As might be expected from these symptoms, fibromyalgia patients suffer from considerable psychosocial impairment and a reduced – in some patients absolutely – ability to work. They also represent a considerable cost to their respective health services as repeat appointments, referrals, hospital admissions, multiple prescriptions and various other therapies are required.

Depending on the diagnostic method employed, prevalence varies from between 1.3 and 8 per cent, and is most common among middle aged women (Smith et al., 2011; Theoharides et al., 2015; Diaz-Piedra et al., 2015). Fibromyalgia is estimated to be between twice and four times as prevalent in females as in males, though it had been reported that in some societies this ratio is even greater (Branco et al., 2010; Lindell et al., 2000; Bartels, 2009). Several epidemiological meta-analyses have demonstrated that fibromyalgia is

3 The link with weather appears to be widespread among patients, but disputed by researchers (see Bossema et al., 2013).

present on every inhabited continent, with inter-country variations ascribed to different clinical attitudes, application of diagnosis, local culture and patient behaviour (Queiroz, 2013).

Comorbidity with other 'functional' (and contested) illnesses is high and it is common for a fibromyalgia patient to also suffer from one or several of the following: chronic fatigue syndrome, irritable bowel syndrome, depression, anxiety, migraine headaches, obsessive compulsive disorder and others, including many multiple non-specific symptoms (Goldenberg et al., 2008; Arnold et al., 2006). In some study populations it has been found that more than half of fibromyalgia patients have seven or more chronic comorbidities (Vincent et al., 2015).[4]

The aetiology and pathogenesis of fibromyalgia remains poorly understood, but it is posited that some combination of genetics, central and automatic nervous system dysfunction, neurotransmitters, hormones, immune system deficiencies, external trauma, environmental factors and psychiatric problems are involved. No one, definitive aetiological narrative has been established and as yet no consistent enough biomarker has been discovered that can indicate and demarcate fibromyalgia with any reliability (Giacomelli et al., 2014). As such, the diagnosis of fibromyalgia remains a process of elimination and subjective reporting, occasionally in tandem with the ACR criteria.

A major problem with identifying fibromyalgia is its similarity to other conditions, and patients often end up being diagnosed with a multitude. A literature review by Aaron and Buchwald highlighted this problem, noting that despite different case definitions, overlap between conditions appeared to be high:

> The existing literature, although dispersed across many disciplines, suggests that many unexplained clinical conditions—for example, the chronic fatigue syndrome, fibromyalgia, and temporomandibular disorder—share demographic, clinical, and psychosocial features, as well as objective findings. In fact, it has been suggested that the diagnosis assigned to patients with one of these illnesses depends more on chief symptom and clinician specialty than on the actual illness.
>
> (Aaron and Buchwald, 2001, p. 868)

Wessely, Sharpe and Nimnuan (1999) previously argued along similar lines, that each medical speciality appeared to have its own 'unexplained' syndrome which, when examined as patient populations, would seem to overlap greatly in terms of both symptoms and treatment strategies.[5] They concluded that the

4 This should be qualified by noting that, increasing as you go up the age scale, multiple comorbidities are common (see Piccirillo et al., 2008), so in this instance it might be sensible to consider the *quality* of the comorbidities rather than their *quantity*.

5 Incidentally, this paper sparked a debate (ongoing) between 'splitters' who believed in the usefulness of divergent diagnoses and 'lumpers' who argued for a broader category which acknowledged the wide overlap (for a recent summary of

classificatory slicing of different functional somatic syndromes was of questionable utility, given the apparent lack of concrete delineating factors. In place of this, they suggested that a dimensional approach might work better, on the understanding that all present subdivisions are attempts to demarcate something which to a great degree is singular: general functional somatic syndrome.

Perhaps predictably, there was a strong reaction to this hypothesis among some members of certain patient communities, rejecting Wessely et al.'s ideas and in some cases resorting to personal attacks and threats. This backlash illuminated another layer of complexity when regarding this issue: once given a diagnosis, sufferers can build up rationalities and explanatory frameworks with which to understand their condition and become in a sense loyal to these descriptions and unwilling to countenance an entirely new and less legitimate sounding disease that they now supposedly have or indeed have had all along (Wessely and White, 2004).

There are, of course, a number of other ideas orbiting fibromyalgia. For example, Yunus (2011) and some other rheumatologists (Fleming and Volcheck, 2015) are of the view that fibromyalgia is best conceptualised and classified as a central sensitivity syndrome (CSS). This is where the central nervous system is hypothesised to exaggerate pain across different bodily systems and generate a number of debilitating symptoms as the body becomes hypersensitive to external stimuli.[6]

These researchers also take a hard line against the language that is used to describe fibromyalgia patients in other fields, and Yunus argues against the firm division of 'disease' and 'illness' along biomedical lines:

> … differentiation between illness and disease is artificial and contrary to patient interest and hampers proper management of CSS conditions, since anything that is not currently viewed as a disease (i.e., does not have structural pathology, e.g., inflammation, degeneration, or neoplasm) is viewed as predominantly or exclusively psychological and benign and is not taken seriously by the healthcare providers, accentuating the suffering of the patients. In an irresponsible way, this untruthful 'dogma' is passed down from the professor or the attending to the students, and the victims are our patients.
>
> (Yunus, 2011, pp. 1–2)

Elsewhere he has stated: 'Patient-blaming terms like somatization, somatizer and catastrophizing should be avoided' (Yunus, 2015, p. 70).

Regardless of the validity of their physiological explanations, and I don't think I am in a position to pass judgement on that, Yunus and others like him

these arguments, see Lacourt, Houtveen and van Doornen, 2013). It is for this reason – symptom similarity and overlap in populations – that in this section I draw on some chronic fatigue syndrome literature as well as that of fibromyalgia.

6 Hypersensitive in both the allodynic (pain from things which are ordinarily non-painful) and hyperalgesic (when mildly painful things are experienced as excruciating) senses.

recognise a key truth: the way the medical cards are dealt, the cards are stacked against patients with contested illnesses. *Style matters.* The language employed does have strongly negative connotations and the prestige hierarchy of physical and psychological ailments is reinforced (intentionally or not) by its use. These writers are certainly correct to point this out, as well as to note that bracketing 'disease' in the manner that it is, excludes a whole range of conditions from ascending to bona fide disease status with deleterious consequences for the patients involved.

As might be expected, these thoughts are not echoed by all practitioners. Hadler (2003, p. 1669) states firmly that he believes this to be the wrong approach, dismissing central sensitisation specifically as a 'contrived neologism'. The problems faced by patients are largely iatrogenic, he argues, caused by 'treatment acts, dripping with empty promises of elucidation and unproved promises of palliation'. Indeed, Hadler believes that telling patients they suffer from a distinct and diagnosable condition called fibromyalgia amounts to the clinically irresponsible 'medicalisation of misery' and he is not alone in that, or similar, views (for example, Ehrlich, 2003).

Wolfe (2009), for instance, believes that the controversy surrounding fibromyalgia (what he terms the 'fibromyalgia wars') is 'best understood in terms of medicalisation and social construction'. In a later paper, he outlines his position as follows:

> There is as yet no compelling evidence that an underlying central nervous system disturbance contributes in a substantial or clinically meaningful way to the development of fibromyalgia. In addition, neurobiological associations depend on fibromyalgia being a discrete disorder, for which no evidence exists. Even if fibromyalgia is considered to be largely a psychocultural disorder, a strong body of criticism suggests that the definition of fibromyalgia is arbitrary, and the methods of assessment illusory.
>
> (Wolfe and Walitt, 2013, p. 751)

In other words, Wolfe and many doctors across rheumatology and other disciplines believe that fibromyalgia is not a separate clinical entity nor a useful diagnostic tool and its continued existence as a disease concept is the result of social factors and not any underlying medical reality. Furthermore, the insistence on labelling non-distinct, vague symptoms as if they were part of a cohesive whole has the effect of solidifying false illness beliefs, making patients sicker than they were before and impeding potentially effective treatment.

The thinking goes that instead of focusing on coping mechanisms and other aspects of life, patients become 'illness-fixated', reading obsessively about their condition, fastidiously monitoring every spasm and ache, to the point of dysfunction: make illness enough of a part of your life and eventually your life will become illness. Some physicians wonder whether they are even the correct professionals to be dealing with these patients, thinking perhaps that psychologists and social workers might have a better chance at building a beneficial, palliative relationship (Åsbring and Närvänen, 2003).

More adversarially, Malleson (2002) frames his scepticism about fibromyalgia around 'compensation neurosis', the rise in injury payments and what he views as an unscrupulous welfare state that incentivises invalidity. He writes dryly that 'rather than curing diseases, medicine is manufacturing new ones' (ibid., p. 172).

Whether or not we should collect patients with seemingly disparate symptoms under one diagnostic label, or indeed under a series of diagnostic labels, is a difficult question to answer. I certainly have sympathy with those who question its validity as a medical approach. What I do take umbrage with, however, is the suggestion that the 'solution' to this patient population (however they may be composed) is to remove social security benefits and medical nomenclature. My disagreement stems from the fact that, as we shall see, many individuals receive neither welfare payments nor diagnosis for many years, and yet their symptoms persist. These are patients for whom a long-awaited diagnosis comes as a surprise, and for whom the label 'fibromyalgia' is transformational, self-affirming, appearing to reify their distress. Though this initial enchantment with the label can dissipate, as patients more and more come to be underwhelmed by the dearth of information available about fibromyalgia and its lack of cachet as a responsibility-absolving diagnosis, it nonetheless remains true that for many individuals, having a diagnosis is the first stage of building a new identity, one in which they are still ill but where they possess something *specific* as opposed just *something*.

Returning to professional perceptions, on the part of general practitioners and specialists who come into contact with fibromyalgia, survey data is scarce but it would appear to suggest that a majority support a psychosomatic view of the condition.[7] A small minority regard it as a 'non-disease' and some rheumatologists (Kraag, 2002) refuse to receive referrals or provide ongoing care for patients with the diagnosis.[8] Evidence also shows that experienced doctors across a variety of countries lack confidence in diagnosing and treating fibromyalgia, especially in relation to making a differential diagnosis, and that they find fibromyalgia patients frustrating to treat (Walker et al., 1997; Perrot et al., 2012; Homma et al., 2016). A study by Album and Westin (2008) also suggested that doctors regard fibromyalgia as less 'prestigious' than other diseases, placing it bottom of a hierarchy of 38 conditions.[9]

7 A small study of rheumatologists in Canada reported that 55 per cent believed fibromyalgia to be primarily psychosomatic rather than physiological (Ghazan-Shahi, Towheed and Hopman, 2012); another Canadian survey of different specialists reported that with regard to aetiology, 28 per cent thought fibromyalgia was primarily psychological, 23 per cent primarily physiological, 15 per cent psychological and physiological, and 34 per cent were unsure (Busse et al., 2008).

8 Eight per cent of respondents to a *British Medical Journal* survey in 2002 regarded fibromyalgia as a 'non-disease' (BMJ, 2002).

9 This 'prestige hierarchy' was arrived at as follows: 'Respondents were asked to rank these 38 diseases and 23 specialities individually on a scale of 1 (lowest

I could go on, such is the multiplicity of opinion and clinician perspectives that exists on this topic (and indeed related topics), but endlessly mapping the various lines in the sand that have been drawn over the last few decades will simply serve to make the same point over and over again: fibromyalgia is a terribly convoluted and tangled affair.

It is inevitable, I surmise, that such an interwoven conflict of diagnostic reliability, clinical pragmatism and aetiological ambiguity will continue unless wholesale epistemic change is enacted across the medical world and conditions of this sort – subjective, symptomatic – come to be regarded as valid disease entities despite their clear incompatibility with biomedical methods of ratification.[10] Should this change not be forthcoming, and the evidence is that it is slow to do so, then undoubtedly such conflicts will continue.

What is likely, then, is that patients will continue to meet a range of reactions in the clinic. There being, as described above, no completely established 'medical' view, the response that patients receive can be incredibly diverse. The most damaging of these from the patient's perspective is that of disbelief or suspicion. As Harth has written:

> … patients with fibromyalgia have to shoulder a burden seldom borne by individuals with other medical conditions. Fibromyalgia sufferers are frequently not perceived as having a distressing condition … patients with fibromyalgia seeking help from their physicians may encounter hostility, skepticism, confusion and therapeutic nihilism.
>
> (Harth, 2013, p. 64)

Harth also notes that 'their families, their friends and their co-workers are often sceptical of their symptoms or their functional impairment'. This atmosphere of disbelief and the discrediting of an individual as a producer and communicator of knowledge has been analysed from an epistemic perspective by a number of authors, most notably Fricker (2007), under the banner of 'epistemic injustice'.[11] This concept can for our purposes be simplified: it is a state in which a speaker's credibility is diminished or erased due largely to prejudice on

prestige) to 9 (highest prestige), based on how they believed most health personnel would rank them. The wording of the question was for the prestige of diseases (in translation): "Below you will find a list of 38 diseases or disease categories. Please give each disease a number based on the prestige you imagine it has among health personnel. A disease you feel is considered to have a low prestige should be given a low number, the lower the prestige, the lower the number. Oppositely, a disease you feel have a high prestige should be given a high number, the higher the prestige, the higher the number. Please circle the number you choose".'

10 Or, it should be noted, unless the conditions in question can be more successfully assimilated into biomedical structures through the discovery of some underlying pathology.

11 Note that Fricker does not explore the medical aspect of epistemic injustice (see also Hookway, 2010; Coady, 2010).

the part of the listener. Lying at the juncture of epistemology and ethics, epistemic injustice can be used to understand how communication can be stacked for and against certain parties, and the damage that can arise from such arrangements.

Originally, this concept was used to bring attention to the ways in which the gender and race of the speaker, among other irreducible features of a person's identity, might lead to the systematic devaluing of their perspective and the discounting of any epistemic contributions an individual thought or was required to make in a given situation. Recently, however, it has been expanded and applied to medical contexts.

Carel, Blease, Kidd and others have argued that it is especially applicable in healthcare settings, both in regard to the doctor–patient dynamic (the 'encounter') and also to broader issues of medical training and policymaking. Epistemic injustice can result not only in bad interpersonal relations (no-one enjoys being patronised or ignored), but also in the missing or misinterpreting of key information because the epistemically privileged individual has chosen to interpret the experiences of another entirely through a framework that undermines the credibility of the patient's communication.

What should be evident by now is that the fibromyalgia patient reporting debilitating pain is not often afforded the same epistemic status as an individual with, say, gallstone problems would be.[12] That this occurs both in the clinical context and outside, and that it can fluctuate over time in relation to external events ('belief turns to disbelief as when tests come back normal'), is of great interest to us here.[13] Routinely, their self-reporting of symptoms and pleas for sympathy are filtered by doctors and those around them in a manner which diminishes their severity and shifts the moral onus from external dysfunction to individual responsibility once it becomes apparent that their problems stem from fibromyalgia rather than some other, more acceptable source.

It is this, the broad *reaction* to fibromyalgia and all its attendant consequences for individual patients, that will be the focus of this half of the book. In order to flesh out or bring to life some of the conflicts and confusions discussed above, in the next chapter I will present the experiences of three patients. The variation present in their stories will hopefully elucidate some of the more tricky aspects of this subject: their symptoms, the meanings they are given by themselves and others, the bureaucratic and medical pillar-to-posting, the compromised and transformed sense of self and surroundings … These can all be seen most starkly when shown through the lives of real patients.

12 This particular form of epistemic injustice is referred to as 'testimonial'.

13 The quote is from the movie *Voices from the Shadows*, directed by Josh Biggs and Natalie Boulton, also used as an example by Carel (2016b).

Chapter 6

Three patients

In this chapter, I will briefly provide (broadly speaking) case histories of three patients who have been diagnosed with fibromyalgia, starting with Lucy. All names have been changed.

Lucy

Lucy worked for 25 years for what was the Department for Social Security and is now the Department for Work and Pensions, in a job centre, before she was forced to leave due to ill health. Initially, she had been to see her doctor about some lower back pain, but the scans they completed came back negative. Following this, her wrists and hands began to hurt and the doctors suspected that she might have RSI. Then:

> … other bits started aching and being problematic and I was going in quite a lot. The doctors thought it was in my head, that it was depression, that I was feeling low which I wasn't. I was just getting fed up with not being able to do things.

Prior to these complaints, Lucy had led an active life, playing sports and exercising frequently. She felt frustrated by the increasing limitations that her mysterious symptoms were placing her under. Eventually she got a diagnosis:

> I was referred to a chronic pain consultant and he was the one who said it was fibromyalgia, which I'd never heard of. All the key points were hurting and the symptoms fitted in with that. He pieced everything together.

Having a name to put to her symptoms allowed Lucy to conduct research, and past events began to congeal into a coherent illness narrative for her. Recounting her personal history, she placed salience on two traumatic events that occurred within quick succession of each other: a bad car accident that required treatment and divorce from her husband. Lucy now believes that within nine months of these things happening she began to develop pain across her body. The pain itself is bad but she has found ways to manage it. If she has a flare up, it can take a while for the worsened symptoms to return to normal, and though they never leave her entirely, she has developed coping mechanisms which she tries to employ as diligently as possible. Still, it is often a case of simply 'muddling' through.

Since her diagnosis, Lucy's experiences with doctors have not been overly positive. Largely she has found GPs to be unsympathetic, treating her as if she is wasting their time and occasionally inducing guilt on her behalf because of the expense of long-term treatment:

> A GP called me in to up my medication but purely on the basis that it was around twenty pound a box cheaper than the medication I was on. He went through the cost of it and how much I was costing the surgery. You feel like a drain on their resources and blooming angry as well. I didn't actually want to increase my medication but you're just kind of thrown into it.

Feeling pressured in this way was not the only poor communication Lucy had with her doctors. In other instances she struggled to get them to appreciate that she felt she knew her body well enough to act as a competent translator:

> You have to prove yourself all the time and say well yes, this really does hurt. Especially when they say it's depression. I've suffered from depression in the past, I know what it's like and no, *this* is a pain, it's really hurting me. I've had other pains that aren't fibro and I told him it wasn't the same but he said, 'We'll add another tablet in, it must be the fibro.' Trying to distinguish and tell them that no, it's something different, is met with the cop-out that it must all be fibro, off you go, you'll be fine. People just aren't listening to what you're saying and you're just labelled as someone with chronic pain symptoms.

The GP surgery is not the sole location that Lucy found it difficult to get the way that she was feeling across to a professional in a manner that she deemed acceptable. After trying and failing to find further, more flexible employment, she found herself back at the job centre she had left due to sickness, for a disability assessment. She felt that throughout her appraisal she was made to feel as if they regarded her condition as one which could be alleviated through willpower:

> The chap I saw there went on about people who have lost their limbs and how they use their mind to get rid of the phantom limb pain and that. He was sort of implying that it was all in my head and that I should be able to use my mind to control all of these pains. It wasn't until I burst into

> tears and argued back about fibro that he changed his opinion. He still put fibro in inverted commas as if it wasn't a real illness though, which did rather annoy me.

Lucy bristles at the suggestion that her symptoms are in her head – that is to say controllable, somehow invented.[1] She recounts lying in bed, crying in pain and wishing that those people who doubt her could see her, so that they can see the evident distress she is in. 'You try living with this', she says to these people, 'I'm not making it up.'

Despite this anger at her treatment and desire for greater recognition of her discomfort, Lucy tries to maintain a positive outlook, and believes that this assists her in dealing with her symptoms:

> I could be miserable every day if I wanted to be. It doesn't do anyone any help. It doesn't help me to be miserable and dwell on things so that's why I don't want to. It's very easy to be depressed when you're feeling that, really, half of your life has gone and that the person you were before has disappeared. I just want to get on with trying to cope with it.

It is this attitude that she takes with her into a local fibromyalgia support group, of which she is treasurer. Here, too, they try not to dwell and rather focus on sharing palliative solutions and organising events to raise money. Lucy is simultaneously resigned to her fate and taking regular steps to alleviate it, a common bind for chronically ill patients. She doesn't fear that it is fatal, has her own understanding of what the disease means and has altered her life as much as possible to cope with the disjunction it has caused. Samuel's story is quite different.

Samuel

Samuel's symptoms have a distinct starting point: he was attacked from behind in the street in an unprovoked assault. Samuel was 'lucky enough' to pass out quickly, but later was shown CCTV of the attackers striking his head with bottles until they smashed. He was admitted to hospital that night, his 'nose broke, bed covered in blood'. Despite this, when his wife came to see him he checked himself out, not realising the severity of his condition. Within a week he noticed a dramatic deterioration in his motor skills and found himself unable to complete simple tasks like opening the door of his car.

1 There is perhaps some confusion on this point. When medical professions use the terms 'all in your head' or similar, they may well mean to say that the pain is real and that, though the cause is psychological rather than physiological, the patient bears no responsibility for it. However, this is not the way such statements are interpreted by patients, who receive the message as if they have been accused of having agency in relation to their symptoms.

Further tests revealed a massive blood clot, and doctors sought permission from Samuel to write up his case in a journal as they had never before seen such a large clot in that area of the brain in someone still alive. It was successfully removed, but this was not the end of Samuel's problems.

Initially it seemed as if he was on track to make a full recovery. He was able to get a job as a support worker in social care, helping young people with behavioural problems, and he tried to put the attack behind him. In time, however, his symptoms did not disappear but rather began to multiply and worsen. He would get spasms down the left hand side of his spine and at the top of his neck, pains in his legs, was 'fatigued all the time, constantly tired' and 'never seemed to get a proper sleep'. Often, he would 'wake up half an hour after going to sleep, in a cold sweat'. Seizures and memory problems became a reality of daily life that Samuel had to adjust to.

He found the response from the GP unhelpful. They prescribed painkillers, building and diversifying the dose until he felt that his house was 'like a chemist' but doing little to alleviate his symptoms. 'All they do is give you tablets,' he said, 'medicate, medicate, medicate.' The problems he reported were also met with scepticism:

> My GP told me that if I ignored it, it would go away. And that they didn't believe in fibromyalgia. I said 'Well, the pain I'm in … I'm not imagining the pain.' I wasn't getting anywhere with him and it was really depressing me. I'm in so much pain and the doctors were telling me to just ignore it.

It became hard at times for Samuel to distinguish between which symptoms were emanating from his body and which were being induced by the significant amount of medication he was taking. Night tremors interrupted his sleep even more, and he became increasingly light-sensitive and resorted to keeping the blinds down in his house so that he could get some relief. In response to the latter of these problems, he now wears glasses with an anti-glare coating to afford him a little respite from bright light. Both of these symptoms he initially put down to the drugs he had been prescribed, but finds it understandably difficult to untangle causality in a body so racked by strange symptoms and ingesting so many painkillers.

He also started having frequent seizures. The following situation might make clear the frightening and disorienting nature of Samuel's condition:

> I was in the house when I woke up and I was covered in sweat and I don't know if I'd had a seizure or what happened but I'd run up the stairs to the toilet and the next thing I know I'd woke up on the floor and I'd banged my head and I had massive lumps on both sides. I had a temperature but I don't know how it happened. I'd also urinated when I'd collapsed up the stairs.

While at work he suffered another seizure and had to take a fortnight off, during which time he remained mostly on the sofa, only rising to use the bathroom. His symptoms during this time accord with what many fibromyalgia patients refer to as a 'flare up': his 'muscles were agony all over … like [he'd] been beaten'. He was able to return to work but lost his driving licence as a result of the seizure.

This was to prove costly, as his employment then deemed him to have frustrated his contract as a result of becoming unable to drive. Not able to work, at least in the short term, he decided to apply for a Personal Independence Payment, which involved an hour and a half drive to the nearest centre:

> My wife was taking me. They were asking me questions like, 'How did you get here?', to which I said, 'My wife drove me.' Then asking me if I could count, asking me to spell things backwards. I actually got it wrong, and then I got confused and then eventually got it right. They were asking me, 'If you paid a pound …' and all these questions about the change. These were the kinds of questions they were asking me. I told them about my symptoms. I had the doctor's report, the neurologist's report, my rheumatology report. When I got home I got a letter saying basically I got zero points altogether, that I had made my way there using map-reading, that there was nothing wrong with me and that I was fit to work.

Samuel noted with dark irony that though he was declared fit to work by the authorities, it was essentially on health grounds that he had become unemployed in the first place. His desire to work has not been diminished, but he feels the stigma of the job centre:

> They look on it like you don't want to work. I do want to work, I want a normal life. I don't want to be in the house the whole time, I want to go out and provide for my family.

Samuel's experiences are a harrowing example of the transformational nature of disease. His life has been, perhaps permanently, altered beyond recognition. Before he was attacked he worked two jobs and described himself as 'constantly active, very fit', with a 'positive outlook on life'. He has gone from being 'a really happy person' to one in the grips of despair, unsure of where to look for help and what steps to take towards recovery. 'It's got to the stage now', he says, 'where I'm unemployed, not entitled to anything … I don't know where to turn. With the income coming into the household, I'm basically just above the breadline.'

Clearly, multiple anxieties converge upon a case such as Samuel's: the frustrated ambitions of modestly providing for and raising a family and putting food on the table alongside a life now constricted and squeezed by medical realities, all the time in the shadow of mysterious and humiliating symptoms.

Samuel has found that singing in the choir his sister runs alleviates his problems, if only for a short time. When he sings, he feels the muscles in his back relax, and the pain leaves his body momentarily. Typical of the explanatory void in which fibromyalgia patients must live their lives, he is unsure of why or how this happens, but glad that it does.

Lauren

Lauren's experience is more ordinary than Samuel's, but her life no less reconstituted by illness. Her introduction to the condition was more gradual, as she found herself repeatedly getting ill without explanation or proper recovery. She contracted a serious chest infection that lasted for four months, and from there the symptoms worsened and spread, despite the use of steroids and antibiotics. Lauren began to hassle the doctors, telling them that she believed the pain was getting more severe: she was getting aches in her lower back and her right arm and shoulder seemed permanently sore. As she explains, it was hard work getting a referral:

> It was a constant badgering, going to the doctors every week and saying I feel really ill. Nothing seemed to fit the pain. He'd done the blood tests and everything. Nothing came back, it was all clear. It took two years to get him to let me see somebody.

In the end, she was sent to see a rheumatologist, who diagnosed her within ten minutes as having fibromyalgia, giving her a name if not a complete explanation for what she was going through.

Lauren's experience here is fairly standard of the patients I interviewed, and it offers clues as to why some doctors dread dealing with fibromyalgia patients. She's clearly in pain, but the pain is widespread, non-specific and non-observable. The GPs think that they know what she is going to say before she comes in the door: that this hurts and that hurts and why can't they do something about it? No doubt the medical professional feels somewhat helpless to aid such patients, who in turn feel frustrated that it seems as if the doctors are ignoring or downplaying their symptoms. Lauren recognises the difficulties faced by doctors, and shares in their frustrating ignorance: 'They just don't know what to do. They have no knowledge of fibromyalgia, and that's the hardest part.'

Once she got a diagnosis and learnt a little more about the condition through personal research, Lauren thought back through her life and began to see a clear pattern of tiredness, pain and infections. She now believes that these problems stemmed directly from sexual abuse she suffered as a child at the hands of her brothers and brother-in-law. We can see here what Hacking means when he talks about 'making up people': before her diagnosis, Lauren had been the victim of abuse as a child and then subsequently yet separately lived a life frequently interrupted by illness, which culminated in her lengthy chest infection and the search for its explanation. Now, diagnosis in hand, she is able to make sense of her personal history in a new way, and events in her life that previously were explained away or forgotten clot around a new, all-encompassing explanation. This is not to say that in some way that her beliefs are incorrect, it is just to say that before she became aware of the category fibromyalgia, the inferences and connections she now draws between things that have happened to her had no soil in which to grow.

However, there were still times she doubted her label. Mostly this was due to the multifaceted nature of what she was experiencing: how could all these symptoms belong to the same thing? 'The pain was in my shoulders,' she said, 'down my neck, down my back, everywhere. And I was incontinent. I thought, "This can't just be fibromyalgia." But that's what I was told, that there are many elements to it. And that's how it works.'

The pain became so much of an issue for Lauren that she had to give up work. She was always someone who worked, sometimes up to three jobs at the same time, and this change of lifestyle has been hard to swallow. Lauren talks of an utter transformation:

> It's just changed me completely. I'm stuck in the house. I go out twice a week for shopping and that's it. I'm not the person I used to be at all. It has forced me into something, somebody that I'm not. And it's very difficult when you've always been an active person. I feel like I'm missing out on life. People see me and think 'She looks well', but they really don't know what's going on inside. I come home and cry for no reason. I sit and cry and there's no reason whatsoever for it.

Lauren's is not the only life left unrecognisable by her condition. Her husband, Gary, has become not just a partner but a full-time carer. He says 'I basically don't know who I'm going to get when I come home. There's no social life. And basically she's always …' His voice trails off before he says, 'she tends to require me all the time'.

Gary admits that he was sceptical for some time about his wife's health issues. 'It took me about twelve months', he says, 'to get over the idea that she was faking it. It was very difficult to understand the illness.' Now, though, he recognises in his wife a genuine dysfunction, and his concern is to care for her and to assist her in getting recognition and support from the state. He has been disappointed by what he views as the cynical attitude of those who determine whether or not she is eligible for social security payments:

> It took a long time to get disability allowance and even now we're getting home visits basically looking at ways of taking money off her. You only have to tell someone who comes to visit that you can walk so many feet and they'll take the money off you. Before this happened, I always

> thought it would be your worst-case scenarios that they would take into account.

I do not wish to analyse these cases too deeply, as every individual has a different experience. Instead, I have drawn these three vignettes for the simple purpose of adding flesh and sinew to the dry bones of aetiology, diagnosis and pathogenesis, in order to show some of the ways in which theoretical conflicts and ambiguities play out in the lives of those in pain. Even from the short overview presented here of Lucy, Samuel and Lauren we can appreciate the complexity and frustration present in fibromyalgia, both on the part of the patient and on that of the doctor. We can also see clearly that the arguments about diagnosis are not baseless, and that establishing a *positive* manner of diagnosing is nearly impossible at present. This is evident from the stories I have presented above: Samuel and Lauren are quite different in symptomatic presentation and the series of events that led to their problems are far removed, yet they still received the same diagnosis. It would seem fair to say that they have both received diagnoses of exclusion. Evident too is the swirling cloud of validation, legitimacy, stigma and epistemic injustice that seems to surround fibromyalgia patients: each of the three talked of being disbelieved, being suspected, being talked down to.

All of the examples presented above could be classified under Frank's scheme as 'chaos' narratives, stories of individuals who have lost faith in the direction or narrative substance of their condition, who begin to see no end to their symptoms. These individuals try to live day by day rather than indulge in thoughts of recovery, not because they would not like to recover but because they see little evidence to suggest that they will.

Now that I have sketched an outline of the clinical picture and provided a sample of the some of the ways in which this condition intersects with patient's lives and identities, we will turn to *pain*, both as a primary symptom and a locus for miscommunication, disbelief, and the everyday drudgery of living in severe discomfort.

For the remainder of this book I will draw upon conversations I have had with patients, using their words – as I have above – to illuminate a point I wish to make. These individuals were drawn from the UK, and though they provided me with much food for thought, I do not intend their words to be the focus of the study itself here. They are more adornments, ways of saying the same thing in a situated, less abstracted manner. They are not representative, because they cannot be; they belong to individuals, not archetypes. I use them in an unashamedly selective way, to try, as I said, to give life to the theorising, and to show what it means to a person, in their own words, to be disenfranchised and delegitimised, and stigmatised and depressed and disbelieved, to find themselves *changed*, in other words, by the world around them as reconfigured by illness.

Chapter 7

Pain

Introduction

If there is one central symptomatic locus of fibromyalgia, it is pain. Underlying the headaches, interrupted sleep and forgotten words on the tips of tongues is the near-constant presence of bodily discomfort – aching muscles and searing joints, and in this section I would like to examine this amorphous problem from a philosophical viewpoint. Pain is an archetypical example in discussions of solipsism, assessing the existence of internal states, scepticism about private language and the like and indeed, the philosophical tradition of pain goes back millennia. What I would like to bring attention to in this section, however, is the specific problems that pain in contested illnesses poses in contemporary settings.[1]

It strikes me that the questions we should ask of pain in relation to fibromyalgia are the following: how do patients describe and communicate their pain? Does this tell us what the pain is *like* or something else? What is our reaction to the pain, as in, why the air of scepticism and the apparent downplaying of severity? Where do we think the pain comes from and why is this important? And how do these questions relate to each other? The problem of pain as it relates to fibromyalgia is about belief and the conflict between medical and subjective methods of communicating information about the body, but it is also a problem about how the body communicates information

1 I am not alone in thinking this is a pressing concern. Rita Charon said in 2016 that 'unremitting pain is … our contemporary central dilemma' (quoted in Padfield and Zakrewska, 2017); on a side note, an interesting question for which we do not have the space to consider: in light of what has been discussed thus far in relation to identity and the socially influenced mediation of experience, can we discuss pain as a historically consistent entity? In the same way in which an identical act five hundred years apart (say, having sex with a man) is rendered fundamentally different by the social architecture which structures our interpretations, memory and indeed experiences of events, could it not be said that the pain Montaigne or Epictetus endured was somehow a distinct object from that which I feel when I stub my toe? Or have is there something more fundamental to pain that no amount of social mediation can change?

about itself. Why don't we look at a fibromyalgia patient and see a person in pain in the same way we do of someone wounded or sick in other ways?

Excruciating, omnipresent pain

I doubt greatly that many fibromyalgia patients would take issue with René Leriche's description of pain as an object which is 'always purposeless' (quoted in Buytendijk, 1971, p. 161). Certainly, it is something they could do without.[2] Two factors converge in the descriptions of pain that I have heard or read from patients: its excruciating severity and its omnipresence. Painkillers, lifestyle changes and meticulous planning all appeared to help individuals moderate the symptom but none would eliminate it entirely. Many spoke of the pain pulsing through their bodies 24 hours a day, seven days a week, and the metaphors that some chose to use to illustrate their experiences speak of a group of people who firmly believe that what they are going through is without precedent in their pre-illness lives:

- 'What's the pain like? Gnawing. It's constant. It's always there. It's kinda part of … I say it's part of who I am now.'
- 'What I can only describe as, it feels like, if someone put a candle under your skin. It feels like you're almost on fire from inside. I know it's weird describing it like that but that's kind of what it feels like, that you're actually burning from the inside out. It's everywhere, it never goes.'
- 'If someone said to me there was a pain like it I would have possibly told them it's not true. Well you know what, there is pain like it. It's horrible.'

This symptomatic profile has a limiting effect on people's lives. That is to say, it reshapes what they are able to do on a day to day basis, but also on how they plan for their future. Chronic pain and its treatment seeps into many different aspects of a person's life and changes the way they view possibilities. One patient, for example, spoke frankly about the fear that her symptoms might restrict her ability to raise children:

> I don't know if I could have children. I'm sure I could physically, as far as I know I'm fertile and stuff, but could I come off my medication for nine months? Because I can't take the stuff I'm taking while pregnant, it's dangerous. I'd have to come off that. And then lifting the child … if I do that it only makes it worse the next day and make the tiredness really

2 Though perhaps not completely. Patients with a total inability to feel pain (congenital insensitivity to pain with anhidrosis) very often live difficult, truncated lives, and even regional insensitivity to pain can cause serious problems, as in peripheral diabetic neuropathy, where amputation after the fact is often not enough to save patients' lives (see Daneshjou, Jafareih and Raaeskarami, 2012; Pendsey, 2010).

> bad. Because you need to physically look after a child … You can't just lie in bed all day if you've got kids.

When I listen to patients or read their accounts of the symptoms they experience, I often think of the poverty of language in relation to pain and fibromyalgia. It is this deficit, this difficulty in expression, which we will turn to now.

Communicating pain

The trouble of conveying pain has, of course, famously been explored before, but it did not lead me in this instance to think about beetles in boxes. Or, at least, not straight away. I was first drawn towards the question of legitimacy in pain being a straightforward issue of inadequate communication.[3] If patients could not translate their pain into accessible forms for others, would this go some way to explaining the lack of compassion they complain of routinely receiving?

Certainly, a lot of the patients I have spoken with suggested that unless you had the condition yourself, you would never truly understand what it felt like. 'Only people with the condition', said one patient, 'can understand how somebody feels'. 'People don't understand what it's like', said another, 'they don't understand the amount of pain'.

Of course fibromyalgia patients are far from being the only ones who have issues communicating their symptoms. Many people with different conditions have likewise found the tools available to them inadequate for the task of getting others to understand how it is they are feeling.

Throughout the 1990s, Mark Collen suffered immense and chronic pain after herniating a disk in his lower back, causing long term nerve damage. He struggled to articulate how he was feeling to his practitioner and felt that the vision of true pain which he held both in his head and, against his will, in his back was obscured behind a clunky and inexpressive linguistic medium. In desperation, he turned to art as a method of conveying his symptoms visually. This form of representation actually improved the treatment he received as the doctors felt they better understood what was happening in Mark's body and how it was making him feel. Buoyed by this success, he founded The Pain Exhibit at the turn of the new millennium, an online collection of artworks produced by those in pain. It aims to educate healthcare providers and the general public as to the unspoken and unspeakable nature of some illnesses. Though a fair number of them are harrowing, what is more striking is the directness with which they portray pain. These are not allusions to hidden disquiet, they are visceral demonstrations of agony, and they illustrate more

3 Rather than a grander problem of language itself, *à la* Wittgenstein (see Wittgenstein, 2009).

than anything the penury of language when it comes to describing physical misery.

Spurred on by this work and others, researchers since have tried to test the utility of using non-verbal communication tools in clinical settings, mostly through the employment of visual aids developed in conjunction with patients. The success of such approaches has been mixed, but what is clear is that the work engages with the same problem: we struggle to talk about pain in a way that other people understand (Main, 2014; Padfield, Zakrzewska and Williams, 2015).

Virginia Woolf (2002) decried this exact issue nearly a century ago. 'English', she stated, 'has all grown one way': towards romance and psychology and schemes, greed and jealousy, power and attraction. Little attention is given to the body, which 'all day, all night ... intervenes'. Indeed, 'the merest school girl, when she falls in love, has Shakespeare, Donne, Keats to speak her mind for her; but let a sufferer try to describe a pain in his head to a doctor and language at once runs dry'. It would appear that we have not expanded our means of expression sufficiently in the years since.[4]

For writers like Scarry (1985), it is not illness in general but pain specifically where our language is unable to bear the load placed upon it (see also Neilson, 2016). There is a fissure between the irrepressible veracity of being in pain and the detached uncertainty of viewing others in apparently similar situations. As she writes: 'to have pain is to have certainty; to hear about pain is to have doubt' (Scarry, 1985, p. 13).

Part of this doubt comes from the bluntness or inappropriateness of the tools we employ. Scarry takes particular issue with the metaphors commonly used by those in pain, and splits them into two types. Patients, she says, talk of either an 'external agent' or of 'bodily damage'. The former frames pain in imagery of attack from or damage sustained as a result of something coming from outside: a hammer, a drill, a knife, a flame. The latter discusses pain in terms of broken bones, twisted muscles, aching organs. Neither of these approaches, argues Scarry, provide the listener with an 'identical' description of pain. They are rather referents or associative images that approximate a non-referential process. That is to say, their use separates our vision and understanding of the pain from the pain itself: we visualise the hammer or the broken bone rather than placing the pain in its actual context.

This being true, it is still possible to impart a portion of our physical experience to others through imagery; we are not entirely impoverished linguistically, and I am in no doubt that the more articulate among us can paint

4 It is not just a problem of the English language, either. Canguilhem writes (in French): 'It is impossible for the physician, starting from the accounts of sick men, to understand the experience lived by the sick man, for what sick men express in ordinary concepts is not directly their experience but their interpretation of an experience for which they have been deprived of adequate concepts' (Canguilhem, 1991, p. 115).

vivid pictures of their interior landscapes. Certainly I can think of many memorable descriptions of pain in fiction, such as the following by John Updike (who so often wrote beautifully on pain) in his novel *The Centaur*:

> By searching through his body he can uncover any colour and shape of pain he wants: the saccharine needle of the toothache, the dull comfortable pinch of his truss, the restless poison shredding in his bowels, the remote irritation of a turned toenail gnawing the toe squeezed beside it in the shoe, the little throb above his nose from having used his eyes too hard in the last hour, and the associated but different ache along the top of his skull, like the soreness left by his old leather football helmet after a battering scrimmage down in the Lake Stadium.
>
> (Updike, 1970, p. 180)

Or Lorrie Moore's wonderfully succinct and evocative portrait of a headache: 'sometimes the zigzag of a migraine made its way into her skull and sat like a cheap, crazy tie in her eye' (Moore, 2008, p. 164).

Even if we admit that pain is ultimately incommunicable, it is not clear why using metaphors and imagery such as in the passages above that allow us at least an indication of what another person is going through is worse than giving up on the idea of communication at all. In a clinical setting, throwing your hands up and stating that pain speaks in an inaccessible language and therefore not worthy of effort is a non-starter.

Many patients have little problem putting their problems into words, and often refrain from using metaphors at all: they talk about pain as something self-evident and are more interested in communicating its reach – both across their bodies and across their lives. What I am trying to say by all this, however circuitously, is that it is not the inherent deficiency of language that leads to miscommunication or scepticism in relation to fibromyalgia patients' pain. Their ability to describe what they are going through in words is just as adequate as a non-specialist with cancer, and so the suspicion – and I think suspicion is the right word here – that they are being misleading, or exaggerating, or misunderstanding what their body is telling them, must come from somewhere else.

Non-verbal communication and the limits of empathy

An important and obvious point to raise at this stage is the fact that pain is communicated by more than just language. The state of being in pain is expressed to and understood by others not just, or even most often, through words but by means of 'serialised bits of pain behaviour – grimacing lips, wincing eyes, moans issuing from the larynx, writhing torsos, and so on' (Schrag, 1982, p. 117). It is because of this visual, physical performance of pain that we nonetheless understand when children or animals who cannot tell us how they feel are hurt in some way. Fibromyalgia patients talk about crying with pain, about rolling into a ball, about being unable to stand for a few minutes because of the intensity of feeling, but they also discuss covering up their symptoms, wearing a mask in front of others and finding ways of dealing with what their body is telling them without showing it.

Could part of the problem be not to do with communication per se, but the precise method and manner in which these patients were trying to express themselves? For most people extreme pain has an immediacy to it – a broken leg cannot be ignored, individuals stung by a box jellyfish cannot talk calmly, etc. – but patients I have spoken with personally were able to hold cogent and involved conversations with me, some lasting upwards of an hour, in spite of what they described as debilitating, extraordinary discomfort. I do not wish to be misunderstood on this point: I am not casting doubt on their testimony, but rather questioning to what extent our acceptance of another's pain lies in the way in which it is conveyed. For the worst pain, people around the patient seem to need more evidence than to be simply told *it is the worst*. They need to see that it is the worst, and to understand how it came about. Our powers of empathy do not exist in an explanatory void.

This is a problem which has been identified before in relation to psychosomatic illnesses. It was noted that despite being paralysed or bedridden or suffering some other unfortunate fate, patients often seemed unperturbed by their situation, almost cheerful to be wheelchair-bound or paralysed. This surprisingly care-free reaction was regarded as a strong indicator that the symptoms had no identifiable biological base, and was known as '*la belle indifference*', or, literally, 'the beautiful indifference' (Stone et al., 2006).

I cannot help but be reminded of my experiences speaking with some young doctors in Australia. We were sitting in a pub garden under the Melbourne sun and talk had turned to my research. I was keen to hear what their experience with fibromyalgia had been, given that they worked in various parts of a hospital rather than a surgery and so occasionally saw patients with fibromyalgia brought in from A&E. One of them told me that the typical fibromyalgia patient they'd see would be a woman who appeared normal and might be playing on their phone or reading. Upon admission they would inform the medical staff that they were in excruciating pain, that everything hurt and that they were ten on the pain scale. Throughout, the patient would seem fairly calm and unperturbed. Finally, they would ask for painkillers. Some of the other doctors nodded or laughed in agreement at this portrayal.

No doubt this is a caricature, perhaps exaggerated by the presence of a crowd and a few Victoria Bitters, and a portrait which fibromyalgia patients themselves would wince at (doctors too perhaps), but it illustrates my point: it is not enough to *say* you are in pain in order for that pain to be recognised. This doctor's scepticism, in large part, was founded upon the discrepancy between the pain being reported by the patient and the corresponding enactment of that pain; he simply did not believe that someone who rated themselves that highly on the pain scale would be able to maintain a conversation, entertain themselves on a phone and generally continue to function. To put this in perspective, to report yourself as suffering from that level of pain is to put yourself in a category of distress 'so intense you feel you will go unconscious shortly'.

There may be a biological component to this. Much neurological research has been conducted over the last decade or so which demonstrates that the human brain reacts differently depending on whether it is empathising with another person in an embodied sense, that is to say an individual vicariously shares the emotional sensations of another, or whether the interaction is based upon 'cognitive perspective taking', or a process of reasoning about the intentions, thoughts, feelings and beliefs of another person (Hein and Singer, 2008).

Interestingly, when *empathising intuitively* with a person in pain, many of the same parts of the brain show activity as when we are in pain ourselves (Betti and Aglioti, 2016). This is why it is difficult, especially in person, to witness the distress of another individual or even an animal. Often we find ourselves involuntarily turning away or feeling uncomfortable, or else gripped by a rising urge to help or allay their pain if we can. However, when reasoning about a person in pain, taking their cognitive perspective as it were, different areas of the brain light up.

What this suggests is that there is a biological element to empathy, and that this is activated visually and automatically. Could it be possible, then, that in the case of fibromyalgia patients, the disconcerting (from the perspective of the viewer) lack of visible anguish works against them in terms of gaining sympathy?[5] And that this lack of sympathy, or diminished empathy, detracts from the legitimacy of their pain subconsciously in the minds of those around them?

Fibromyalgia patients complain frequently that others do not see them on the bad days – as during flare ups or other bad periods they did not leave the house, go to work or attend doctor's appointments – and thus get a distorted view of how much they appear to be in pain. Even when out of the house, so to speak, they try to hide what they are going through in order to make their lives easier. As one patient puts it:

> You learn to wear a mask. When people are crossing the street and they say 'oh good morning, how are you?', the answer is 'fine thank you, how are you?' and everyone goes their own way. Nobody actually wants to know the answer to their question. It's a nicety.

Another sufferer had come to the conclusion that fibromyalgia is too complicated and confusing to explain every time they met someone new:

5 It has long been noted in disability studies that lay reactions to different disabilities rely upon contextual and visual knowledge (i.e. how much the dysfunction 'stands out', the meanings surrounding it and how it is encountered). For examples, see Wright (1988) and Schmelkin (1988).

> I've given up trying to tell people what I have, I just say I'm fine. It's difficult to explain how it's had such an immense effect on my life and I don't think anybody could understand that.

Is it possible that all these problems of communication stem from the same place, I wonder? Is it that the pain felt by fibromyalgia patients is somehow different from 'ordinary' pain and therefore necessarily divergent too in its interior presentation? Would this not make it both harder to express and less easy to recognise? Are there different types of pain?

Different types of pain

People without medical or scientific backgrounds tend to have a singular notion of pain: that it has many adjectives but belongs to just one category. Pain can be gnawing, biting, aching, shooting, etc., but there is no Pain A and Pain B. Physiologically, this is incorrect. Pain experts have for some time distinguished between nociceptive, inflammatory, neuropathic and functional pain. Nociceptive discomfort is pain as a nervous response to injury, a message sent through the body as a result of injury, inflammatory pain that which comes after – the lingering pain of tissue damage; neuropathic pain appears to be a malfunction of the nervous system, and functional pain is best framed as distress in the absence of any injury or lesion at all (Dusenbery, 2018). Where nociceptive and inflammatory pain are usually time limited and easily alleviated, their neuropathic and functional brothers are less easily contained, often persisting over many years and proving resistant to treatment.

Fibromyalgia patients do not show any measurable signs of pain, and, as stated above, there is a distinct lack of biomarkers in relation to their condition. Davis and Vanderah (2016) argued that the reason for this is because fibromyalgia patients suffer from a different type of pain than those we are used to looking for. They suggest that traumatic experiences, especially those that occur when we are young, can rewrite our nervous systems and make us susceptible to exaggerated pain responses in later life without corresponding tissue damage. Furthermore, they hypothesise that clinical attitudes towards pain which view it as strictly nociceptive or neuropathic, actively harm the doctor patient relationship in instances such as fibromyalgia. I would extend this point to more general reactions to pain: pain without tissue damage, organ dysfunction, inflammation or bruising is harder to understand and harder to believe.

It is also harder to treat. A varied back-bar of opioids, anti-depressants, anti-inflammatories, muscle relaxants and sleep medicines are prescribed to patients, normally on a tailored, trial-and-error basis. Of the three drugs that are FDA-approved, pregabalin (marketed as Lyrica), duloxetine (sold as Cymbalta) and milnacipran (Ixel, Savella, Dalcipran, Toledomin), two are SNRIs also used to treat depression and similar disorders, and one is an antiepileptic drug.[6] None of the three has been found to treat patients with great consistency or efficacy, and many patients regularly take large doses of each without witnessing a corresponding drop in symptom severity.[7]

How this relates to the notion of pain, or of differentiating within pain, is down to the fact that individuals have an expectation that medicine will be able to reduce suffering in almost all cases:

> My dad died of a cancerous tumour and my aunt died of bowel cancer, and I remember being told that they would never have to be in pain. Nobody had to be in pain. So why is it I have to live in constant pain and nothing can stop that pain? I find that hard to get my head round.

The fact that painkillers that work so well for other instances of pain fail to have a similar effect on the symptoms of fibromyalgia patients serves to increase the feeling of isolation and alienation on their behalf in regard to their bodies, the simple question being that if this were *normal* pain, then surely it would be subject to the same physiological laws and treatable by the same drugs?

To collect the pieces thrown out so far in this section and begin to assemble them, it seems we can say the following. Fibromyalgia patients have problems in the linguistic communication of their pain, but there is no reason that their problems would any more severe than some other conditions. It may be that physical presentation is an issue, in that fibromyalgia patients don't look like they are ill, or like they are in as much pain as they say they are. This is compounded by what could be called their invisibility, the fact that many of them do not seek company or leave the house on their 'bad' days, and by the biological evidence that visual cues are necessary for deep empathy. Furthermore, this might be in part elucidated by the *strangeness* of the pain felt, suggesting a wholly different bodily process. However, there is a further avenue to be explored, that of explanation. The pain that fibromyalgia patients feel exists in an explanatory vacuum. I believe it to be true that, however rudimentary and unscientific, other people generally require some coherent account of the pain in order to recognise it as legitimate.

Recognising the pain of others

When I use the word 'recognise' to talk about pain, I do it quite deliberately. Encountering the pain of a fibromyalgia patient is like meeting someone you think you recognise from somewhere but don't; you ask them

6 SNRI stands for serotonin-norepinephrine reuptake inhibitor. They are a class of anti-depressant drugs commonly used to treat depression and similar conditions.

7 They appear to work on a limited and piecemeal basis, proving marginally effective for a minority of patients (Theoharides et al., 2015).

if they went to this school or used to drink in that pub, and when the answers come back negative you conclude that in fact you do not know this person. We ask: is it something to do with your muscles then? Did they find a problem with your spine? Do you need an operation? And when the answers come back we find ourselves looking at something unknown and therefore fill in the explanatory void with other inferences. We do not know this pain.

Given the difference between automatic empathy and cognitive perspective taking, is it not reasonable for individuals considering the fibromyalgia patient, on the basis of their presentation, to downplay their symptoms for good reasons? In that, having put themselves 'in the shoes' of a fibromyalgia patient, they have concluded that, on the balance of evidence, it is more likely that patients are not in fact feeling pain at all. Certainly some individuals do feel like this, and patients speak frequently about coming up against the attitude that what they relaying about their subjective state is subservient to the lack of 'objective' markers of debilitation.

I would like to raise another point, or rather ask another question: is it possible that some of us believe that fibromyalgia patients *are* in pain, but we disbelieve the pain itself? To put this another way, is it that we understand and appreciate that a fibromyalgia patient feels pain, but the lack of physiological basis for that pain leads us to think that either that pain is not worthy of the same sympathy as other instances of discomfort or that somehow that pain is 'not real'?

This is a moral standpoint that, if not necessarily explicitly and consciously taken, is definitely *felt* to be taken by many in the eyes of fibromyalgia patients. The dreaded sentence 'it's all in your head' is repeated frequently by patients as the epitome of dismissiveness and non-empathy: the implication being that though they may well be feeling pain, that pain was self-generated, an internal creation rather than an external threat and, most of all, controllable.[8] In other words, because of the lack of an explanatory framework, their pain is not as worthy as other forms of pain:

> My neurosurgeon, who did my spinal surgeries, when I was still having so much pain after the last surgery, he was basically telling me it was all in my head and that the X-ray and MRI look like they should and so I'm basically just imagining it and remembering the pain I was in.

8 Incidentally, this phrase was used as the title of Suzanne O'Sullivan's 2015 Wellcome Book Prize-winning work, later republished, bizarrely, as *Is it All in Your Head?* The subtitle – *True Stories of Imaginary Illness* – remained the same between editions. The pronounced difference between these two titles obscures the central point: diseases can be 'all in your head', your head in this case being a metaphorical repository for unhappiness and, subsequently, a subconscious puppeteer of your body, without it being anything like 'your fault'.

> Some of them don't believe that it actually exists. One of the consultants, he told me it was all in my head. It's very, very difficult. It feels like you're trying to convince them you're ill.

Pain here takes on the quality of being genuine not because it is felt, but because of its origins, legitimacy afforded not in the case of pain being reported, but in the context of how that pain came about and in what ways we can view it. Of course, different people have different reactions to the pain of a fibromyalgia patient, and I am only analysing here a few responses. But there are patterns, certainly, and, however impressionistically, I have touched upon a few above.

I am in pain and I know I am not in pain

There is one further point I would like to make about pain. In Wittgenstein's (2009) much-repeated and much-discussed private language argument, he uses pain as a prime example. He states that there is little difference between saying 'I know I am in pain' and saying 'I am in pain', because it is incoherent to talk about knowledge of interior sensations in the same way they we deal with exterior facts (i.e. investigation, verification, justification, truth etc.). As Schrag (1982, p. 111) puts it, 'knowing that one has a pain in his foot is assuredly quite different from knowing that a fifth of Beefeaters gin is in the liquor cabinet'.

However, I do not believe it to be an outrageous stretch of the imagination to consider the idea that for fibromyalgia patients, the statements 'I know I am in pain' and 'I am in pain' are not straightforwardly identical, and in fact might not be held to be true simultaneously or at least clash in some previously unforeseen way.

Wittgenstein does not think that we can talk about pain in terms of knowing because it is an internal, subjective phenomenon that we simply *feel*: we are either in pain or we are not, and we cannot submit it to the same analysis that we can other pieces of knowledge about the world. This argument is, of course, grammatical rather than metaphysical: it is about how we use language. I do not intend to challenge this view.

Instead, I intend merely to use his arguments about 'knowing' pain as a way of illustrating the doubt felt by patients, who themselves are not outside of the explanatory void viewpoint I suggested above might account for a portion of the scepticism afforded to their symptoms. Certainly, the indication that several patients gave me was that the lack of positive biomarkers, the inability of others to recognise their pain, the attitudes they came up against, led them in some way to doubt that they were feeling pain at all. This is because they treated 'pain' as an object of knowledge in precisely the way which Wittgenstein said it would be nonsensical to do so, as something to be weighed against the evidence, a framework in which subjective feelings could be overruled, as if it were an external artefact rather than something intangibly personal and interior:

> 'I doubted myself, that's exactly what happened. They had me thinking is it really in my head? Have I really got it? I was doubting myself at one point because no-one was listening to me and I was thinking oh surely, they're professionals, they know what they're doing'.
>
> 'I've been to the doctor and said "am I making this up? Why aren't these painkillers working? Is this just all in my head?"'.

This doubt leads a patient to think that what they have *isn't pain*, and thus they might say 'I am in pain' because our language does not provide them with an alternative and appropriate way of expressing their interior sensations – i.e. something that resembles pain enough to be considered but fails to meet some external criteria – while simultaneously and, sincerely, stating that 'I know I am not in pain'.

Goldberg (2017) makes a similar point to this, though he argues that what is occurring is not the simultaneous in pain/not in pain dichotomy that I have drawn above but rather a question of denying the legitimacy of real, irrepressible sensations:

> By visually representing the pathologies inside the human body, the truth of the phenomenon in question can be discerned. But note that it is not merely the physician qua investigator who uses images of the anatomised body to verify the truth of the matter. The pain sufferer himself/herself/themselves also draw on the epistemic power of the correlative pathological object inside the human body. While pain sufferers do not have the luxury of denying the reality of their pain, they can and do deny its legitimacy, thereby internalising the stigma so frequently directed at people in pain.
>
> (Goldberg, 2017, p. 242)

This discussion rests heavily on the thought that pain has become an object which is visible in a shared sense, and that which cannot be seen or leaves no physiological trace must be something else, something not-pain. An analogy would be to say that though we all continue to carry around boxes with a thing we call a 'beetle' in it, as Wittgenstein instructed, we do so in a society with rudimentary X-ray technology (technology that also carries a lot of prestige) which allows us to view blurry scans of other people's beetles. Most correlate roughly with each other, but some seem incongruous, despite their owner's insistence that what is in their box is a beetle like all others. It is these people we begin to distrust, suspecting that they are not in possession of a beetle as we understand it, despite having limited knowledge ourselves. This view roughly correlates to the situation fibromyalgia patients find themselves in, where modern medical apparatus allows us to view the footprints of pain but theirs leaves little trace.

Pain is not the only symptom of fibromyalgia, however. Patients also report cognitive problems with speech and memory, which we will turn to now.

Dyscognition

One of the strangest symptoms of fibromyalgia has been termed 'fibro fog' (Kravitz and Katz, 2015; Ambrose, Gracely and Glass, 2012). Patients describe this phenomenon as a creeping forgetfulness, a vague and unspecific dulling of their brainpower:

- 'What I'd call "fogginess", lack of clarity of thought. I'll go to do something and forget what I was going to do in the first place and end up doing something completely different. It's frustrating.'
- 'Sometimes when I'm cooking, something is in a different pan or in the top oven and I forget about it so it just gets left, or it burns, or we just don't eat it because I forget. So we have two thirds of the meal rather than the whole meal… We had a house fire a couple of years ago because I left something on the cooker and went out.'
- 'My memory is horrendous. I sometimes can't remember something that happened thirty seconds ago. I can't remember the names of people that I've known for twenty years. I look at them and think, I know you, but I can't come up with their name.'

All of this may well read like the ordinary consequences of ageing and perhaps, given a certain angle, evidence of the confirmation bias present in a condition like fibromyalgia. Those of the medicalisation/iatrogenic school of thought would certainly be tempted to argue that the above is symptomatic of what they already know to be true: people with fibromyalgia become ultra-sensitive to what are simply the normal biological effects of time passing. Healthy people forget things, just like healthy people feel tired and healthy people ache. The hypersensitivity to symptoms which lie on a normal spectrum of distress is precisely what is causing the problem in this view: and a tendency to search symptoms online rather than engage with traditional constraints against illness behaviour (such as close family members) serves to exaggerate the meaning of these symptoms further until they metastasise into a full blown 'illness career'. Barsky and Borus (1999, p. 910), in line with this perspective, argue that 'the suffering of these patients is exacerbated by a self-perpetuating, self-validating cycle in which common, endemic, somatic symptoms are incorrectly attributed to serious abnormality, reinforcing the patient's belief that he or she has a serious disease'.

In thinking about this I am reminded of the episode of *Hancock's Half Hour* where Tony Hancock appears in a state of histrionic convalescence, sitting at his kitchen table inhaling Vicks vapour while surrounding by a variety of bottled remedies. Appealing for compassion from his friend Sidney, his concerns are given short shrift:

> Sidney: 'What's the matter, you've got a cold? You want sympathy? Everybody gets colds.'
>
> Tony: 'Not like I get them.'
>
> Sidney: 'Of course they do.'
>
> Tony: 'No they don't. Samples, that's all they get. Me, I get the full output of the entire germ kingdom.'

Besides being perhaps the first recorded instance of 'man-flu', this exchange is also illustrative of the attitudes that fibromyalgia patients sometimes face: that there is nothing especially unique about their symptoms and that what they are feeling are the 'ordinary' aches and pains of life. The implication here is that they, like Tony Hancock, are not truly or at least seriously ill but merely being melodramatic. As one patient says:

> It's very difficult because if somebody asks what's wrong with you, to try and explain what fibromyalgia is you'll be there forever and people don't want to be lectured. So if you say to somebody 'I've got chronic fatigue', their usual reaction is well I get very tired as well and it's frustrating because you need to explain to them that chronic fatigue is not the same as just being tired. Sitting down and having a cup of tea will not fix it.

Fibromyalgia does not only affect the elderly, but also can be found in young and middle aged individuals who we would not expect to have pain or memory symptoms *at all*. The fact that these patients feel they have the same complaints as older sufferers casts doubt on the idea that fibromyalgia is simply hyper-vigilance to the creaky facts of ageing. For example, consider the following, from a woman in her early twenties:

> I get fibro fog, that is awful. It's almost the worst part. You literally become unintelligent, you can't focus on anything long enough to do anything and you just can't get your brain going.

These issues – fibro fog or 'dyscognition' – have attracted increased clinical attention recently, but that is not what I would like to focus on. Instead, I'd like to make the point that cognitive problems, alongside the gamut of other symptoms fibromyalgia patients experience, alienate patients from other people's expectations of a diseased body. Fibro fog and other symptoms, of which there are an incredible multitude, make fibromyalgia patients harder to 'recognise'.

The reason for this again comes down to expectations. When we encounter illness, we (the lay population) expect it to manifest consistently (to our expectations of consistency as it relates to disease). If you have X, we reason from experience, then that means you will get symptoms Y and Z. One fibromyalgia patient, on the other hand, might present with symptoms N, G and B, whereas a different patient shows symptoms C, D and K. The relationship between the symptoms themselves are important too: through the lay knowledge of medicine we pick up over the years, certain complaints cluster together. A pain in the gut and constipation, for instance, or yellow eyes and jaundice, or fever and a runny nose. Less common combinations involving, say, muscle pain, forgetfulness and fluctuating numbness in your right hand, are harder for people to place, harder to recognise, and without a cogent explanation (which with fibromyalgia is rarely forthcoming), harder to believe. This is made all the more difficult when you consider that another fibromyalgia patient might experience different symptoms – what is an observer to make of all this?

In Chapter 6, a large portion of Samuel's complaints regarded seizures, something that very few patients report. One patient might describe violent shaking, another talk about problems with sweating. A female patient I have spoken to even said that pain was not her main complaint. This inconsistency of presentation goes directly against what we would normally expect to see in a disease.[9]

I seem to be making the case, as others have, that fibromyalgia is a hopelessly vague diagnosis, accommodating a large number of individuals with different complaints. But this reasoning itself speaks to our implicit idea of disease. That is to say, as obvious as it is to point out, our entire causal conception of illness is one which privileges consistent outcomes, regardless of whether the explanatory weight is put on mechanistic or probabilistic footing in any particular instance. This makes sense, but it is not a model that fits fibromyalgia patients – or, to strip away their label, *this symptomatic population*. Because here's the crux: take away their diagnosis and these patients would still feel ill, would still appear in doctors' clinics, would still have

9 I am not saying that all diseases are symptomatically consistent: this is patently false. I am talking in terms of expectations – the subtle, subterranean rudders that guide our gaze. In 'recognised' conditions with variant symptoms there are two factors which explain our 'lack of surprise', or in other words two factors that account for divergent complaints not serving to delegitimise a condition. Firstly, though different symptoms may appear in different individuals, these patterns are normally mapped and so a symptom, though not necessary, will be regarded as sufficient for that condition and not unusual. That is to say, though patients may experience any one of a number of complaints, these symptoms will not display the same chaotic randomness that they appear to in fibromyalgia patients. Secondly, an explanatory framework will normally exist which can provide causal links between symptoms and disease in a way that is not possible, or not currently possible, with fibromyalgia.

trouble functioning on a day-to-day basis.[10] They *do* have many of the same problems, in a broad sense, and what matters here is that they are treated by others on the basis of possessing *something unitary*, irrelevant of how fluid that thing is.

There is a final layer of inconsistency to be addressed. Frank (2013; see also Kleinman, 1988; Charmaz, 1993; Bury 2001; Charon, 2008), as discussed at various points above, details the ways in which sick people think about their illnesses narratively. He states that generally speaking we in the West are preoccupied with restitution narratives, those which tell of healthy people struck down by disease but on the road to recovery – a road which is linear and straightforward. Less thought is given, he says, to chaos narratives: stories of illness with no endpoint and little internal consistency. There is no happy ending with a chaos illness narrative because more often than not there is no ending at all.

Quotes like the following illuminate the trouble that patients have making narrative sense of their disease and its symptoms:

> They say 'We'll just up your morphine, that'll get rid of some of your pain' and it will but it just goes round and round. I just think 'Why can't you treat the cause?' They don't seem to know anything about the cause. I feel like they can't do anything apart from up my medication and I don't want to have it up because then it makes me more tired and sleepy. Is this my life? I'm going to constantly climb up on this painkiller regime until … until what? They can't give me any more? And then I just live in pain or … I don't understand it. I'm not sure where it's going.

This sense of unstructured, open-endedness speaks to the experience of fibromyalgia patients and though many individuals find ways of living with their symptoms and redesigning their lives in a way that allows them to function better, the restitution of the body to previous levels of health is rare. But more than just this aspect of their condition is chaotic: their symptoms, varied as they are in form as detailed above, vary also in severity. This is bewildering for patients; for those around them it jars with what they believe disease to be. We do not expect symptoms to simply flit about the body like a child walking at random between rooms of a house, and neither do they generally appear, disappear and then reappear without any apparent (or, at least, proportional)

10 There is no doubt many people who would disagree with this point and contend that if you took away the diagnosis then there would be no disease and patients would be more likely to recover. The basis on which I dismiss this iatrogenic model is simple: patients find that symptoms persist for years, whether or not a diagnosis is arrived at. And even the possession of a diagnosis such as fibromyalgia is, I believe, an underdetermined factor in the generation and maintenance of symptoms as many sufferers recognise its vagueness and imprecision. It is a loose net, for sure, but the fish it trawls were already in the water.

corresponding *reason*.[11] So when we see a person who, one day to the next, appears to oscillate between physical destitution and well-enough-seeming periods of energy and health, we find it difficult to assimilate this information into the biomedical matrix that informs our understanding of disease. It doesn't fit.

Patients recognise that this is a factor in their condition not seeming valid: 'It changes so much, one minute I'm lying dead on the couch, the next minute I'm like "Let's go cook dinner." I think that's got to be hard for them [her family] to deal with.'

This issue – the inconsistency of symptoms – and the way it is handled by doctors, patients and the people around them, will emerge in different forms as we go through the final sections of this book. Along with the other items discussed above with regard to pain, explanation and belief, it can be a key reason why fibromyalgia patients feel delegitimised, and that their symptoms are not as valid as other ill people's. In the next section, I will look at what relationships can tell us about our collective conception of disease and make the case that for many patients the interactions they have with their family, friends and colleagues in relation to their condition are more important in determining their wellbeing than the medical care they receive, something which has been neglected in previous philosophical treatments of disease, which tend to be more focused on concepts as they relate to healthcare and science.

11 For instance, one patient said: 'Some days it might just be one bit, or start in one bit and go round the rest of the body, or I've had days where it's been full on, everywhere, stabbing pains all over.'

Chapter 8

Relationships

Introduction

A large portion of the philosophy of medicine literature focuses on how we should define certain concepts – health and disease being the main players. Implicit (and occasionally explicit) in these discussions is the salience of deferring to medical definitions and usages of terms. On the one hand this is intuitive: all of what we know about disease, biologically, by definition comes from medical science and discussing illness without talking about healthcare or 'medicine' seems deficient. On the other hand, though medical definitions are extremely important and interactions with healthcare providers laced with meaning, doctors are not the only ones who define disease, and whose definitions have an impact on patients.

I am not here talking about the web of interests that often encircles a disease – the pharmaceutical influences, patient advocacy groups, public funding bodies, etc. – but the regular, very ordinary way in which non-medically involved persons make decisions regarding the sick people around them. It strikes me that when patients talk about disbelief, invalidation, malingering and all the rest of it, what they are commonly referring to is the disbelief of their partners, children, neighbours and friends. This scepticism, the scepticism of the 'man in the street', has not been discussed much within philosophical circles. Perhaps this is because it is so messy, so fraught with caveats, so difficult to pin down. Perhaps also because it is considered metaphysically unsophisticated and consequentially unimportant. Or maybe because philosophers consider this to be sociological or anthropological terrain.

My position is different. The views of non-medical individuals are of great importance in relation to contested diseases, and these views are informed by philosophical standpoints about causality, disease and the body, no matter how unconscious or hidden they may be. It is these standpoints I would like to unearth and hold up as important factors in the happiness and coping ability of those of us who suffer from what I have termed contested diseases.

Being seriously ill with almost any sickness compromises you in a multitude of ways: you cannot do some of the things you used to be able to, or you have to do them in a modified way; your symptoms squeeze and constrict what you are able to focus on, minute by minute; the financial costs of healthcare, special arrangements and income lost by jobs you are no longer able to do adds up and constrains the material aspects of your life … the place you live in becomes 'a world of negotiation, of helplessness, of avoidance' (Carel, 2016b, p. 77). But it also compromises *your person.* [1] Chronic illness transforms an individual's self-concept, their idea of who they are and why they are, and the reactions of others in their immediate social environment are important shaping factors in this process. Carel writes:

> Because it alters one's relation to the world, illness can expose not only the limits of human experience but also the biases of an environment. The moment a particular environment ceases to be familiar and becomes hostile, one is required to reflect on that environment.
>
> (Carel, 2013, p. 350)

Here she is talking about a person's physical surroundings – the way in which stairs become truly visible only once we struggle to ascend them – but it is just as apt a description the permanently altered social relations that come with being ill. Likewise, once this change occurs, it becomes easier to see the biases of this particular environment, in this case not uneven surfaces or previously unacknowledged distances but the unconscious systems of appraisal used to weigh up the validity of another's experience as related by them to you. Or, to put it another way, the structures by which we – ordinary, non-medical individuals – establish epistemic credibility in relation to illness become most clear once tested by an unusual, borderline phenomenon. Fibromyalgia is one such case.

Strangers, acquaintances, friends, family

The first thing to say is that, fairly self-evidently, responses to contested illness vary between individuals. There is no one, universal reaction. There are, however, certain themes that emerge and certain features of a fibromyalgia patient that seem to provoke. These are, as might be expected from the above discussion, the inconsistency and strangeness of symptoms, the distance between what is being said by a patient and what they look like, the lack of a plausible-sounding and medically endorsed aetiological explanation and, in light of this, the growth of scepticism and suspicion of malingering, no doubt

1 Many studies have argued that an individual's sense of self is severely altered by chronic, contested illness. For instance, Whitehead's (2006) work showed that patients with chronic fatigue syndrome found their identities completely reconstituted, and Clarke and James (2003) argued that patients expressed a severe loss of self-esteem as a result of their illness.

exaggerated by the ongoing and pejorative public discourse around welfare payments.

It is perhaps not surprising that patients reported that strangers were the most likely to regard their condition as illegitimate. Confrontations sometimes result from fibromyalgia patients simply exercising their rights as disabled individuals:

> I've had stand up rows in carparks before. People go you can't park here and I say why not and they go you're not old enough to have a blue badge or you can't have a sports car and a blue badge. And it's like really, what does disabled look like? They just have a picture in their heads and it's not me.

Often, patients believe the problem not just to be that they do not look 'ill' enough to meet other people's criteria, but that these people only get to see part of their story. They saw them on a good day, or a good part of a day; they were not witness to when they got home and crashed:

> If someone sees you getting out of the car and you've parked in a disabled space and they look at you because you're walking and they have this idea that you have to be about ninety and in a wheelchair. Society judges you because what they don't see is that if I've gone into town and had a little wander around the shops, I'm struggling to get back to the car because I'm absolutely worn out.

These comments get to the heart of what I am trying to say about expectation and recognition and all the coded ways we appraise those around us, and how this intersects with other conceptions we hold, such as those that concern fairness. We are happy to give extra rights, such as a blue badge, to those who we believe deserve it and what's more, *look* as though they deserve it. The old, the frail, the wheelchair-bound. But something in the minds of a lot of people pricks up at the sight of a young, healthy looking person parking in a disabled space. We do not associate what we are seeing with potential ill health and instead reach for another explanation: that this person is trying to game the system, that they are unfairly benefiting from the generosity and kindness of others.

It is not just complete strangers who hold these views. Given more information, the name of the diagnosis, more regular encounters with the patient, we might expect to see a change in perception. But for some people this change does not occur and they remain suspicious of the motivations of fibromyalgia patients. Some speak about the period following their diagnosis, when acquaintances seemed to recede into the background and lengthy friendships faltered. One patient said, 'I did lose most of the friends that I had'; another told me, 'I've known people for more than 30 years and as soon as I became ill they all disappeared.'

It would be wrong to ascribe this shrinking of a patient's world entirely to prejudice. Fibromyalgia, like most chronic illness, restricts an individual's ability to participate as fully in most activities as they did before, and friendships often require effort to maintain. Thus it may be as an unfortunate side-effect of their condition, rather than solely on the basis of stigma, that patients find their social lives dramatically transformed by illness. As the following story demonstrates, even balancing ordinary seeming occurrences such as a night out with taking care of your body can be fraught with difficulty:

> I'm meant to be going out with a girlfriend tonight, out into town, you know, dancing and all the rest of it, and I absolutely love dancing. Now the worst flare-up I ever had was after a hen do, and as you do we stayed out until 5 a.m. and I was wearing big heels and I was in pain so I was actually drinking while taking tramadol which I probably shouldn't have but I did. And so I was fine. But I was sore the next day and it got worse and worse and in the end I was in bed for four days. So now I'm actually scared, I don't want to go out tonight and I've put it on hold, I've just said I don't know if I can, it's hard to say to her that I'm scared of going out dancing because I don't want to be in bed for days. I think if I were to say I'm going to have a month where I just recoup and all the rest of it then I'm sure I'd never go out again. It's like a vicious circle. If you give up then you will just end up staying in all the time.

This story neatly and sadly summarises the dilemma that patients find themselves in: go out and suffer heavily for it or turn down the invitations until eventually they stop being issued. For some, it is just too costly for them to go at all:

> Friends want to go out for birthday parties and stuff, but I don't go any more because I don't know what I'm going to be like. I've been to places and fallen over while I've been there and then can't get up. Life is very limited.

It would seem that in many cases the reduction of a patient's social activity is a mix of both people who were previously friends dissipating and the unfortunate realities of the illness itself.[2] Some groups are better able to make allowances than others. For instance, one patient spoke with me about their experiences with motorsport:

> It was part of my life before. After I discovered I had fibromyalgia, the rest of my friends that weren't in motorsport walked away, apart from

2 The difficulties of maintaining a social life while suffering from fibromyalgia are discussed well by Arnold et al. (2008).

> one person. Motorsport accepted me. It was a case of, I'm too poorly to be allowed trackside, but there were other roles that I could do.

This patient works as an environmental scrutineer who monitors track noise, and thinks she is a good example of how both sides of a post-fibromyalgia relationship can make allowances in order to maintain and build social interactions.

In some cases, however, the situation is not so ambiguous as it may be with friends and strangers. With those closest to us, most often our families, the chance to skirt around issues of belief, to avoid telling a patient 'what you really think', is not always there. Most of us live lives in close quarters, with little room to hide our opinion about certain circumstances. In other words, within a household it is a lot harder to conceal or disguise your feelings, and sometimes this comes to the fore in hard to handle ways. Relationship breakdown and familial estrangement are common fallouts from fibromyalgia. Trying to tease apart the relative weight that beliefs about the illness, the strain of living and looking after a sick person, the financial and social impoverishment that illness can bring and the 'ordinary' collapse of partnerships that can occur in any relationship is a difficult analysis to undertake. It would certainly appear, however, that in many cases the lack of sincere confidence in a fibromyalgia patient's symptoms and motivations leads directly to the fragmentation of previously solid networks. At the extreme end, you find situations like that experienced by this patient:

> I suffered domestic abuse at the hands of my daughter. She didn't believe I had fibromyalgia. She didn't understand that it was a condition that varies. She really did not grasp that my condition can fluctuate. She would tell me, in her words, that I was 'scamming off the government'. She would pin me in the corner of my kitchen, hurling verbal abuse over at me, that I was lying, that it was all in my head, that I was sick in the head and needed to be locked away from normal people.

In other cases it is parents who disbelieve, or partners, but the central points expressed remain the same: doubt that fibromyalgia patients are telling the truth, the sense that they have some degree of control over their health situation and general embarrassment at their condition. For instance, a patient's mother refused to hold her walking stick for her because she was concerned about what others would think while another's daughter said she didn't think her mum was a good role model because she was a 'cripple'. A patient described to me how she hid aspects of her condition from her parents because she was afraid of what they would think:

> They know about the fibro but they won't know I spent a day in bed yesterday, they just don't get it. They don't know about all the Tramadol.

> We just don't really talk about it. Partially it's because they think I'm being a hypochondriac and I made it up.

The pressure placed on a household by something like fibromyalgia can be immense. Partners and children become de facto carers, and the lack of recognition that fibromyalgia has in broader bureaucratic systems means that support from local authorities is often lacking. For example, one teenage daughter who found herself in the position of caring for her mum was offered much and given little:

> We had a child support officer come round and they promised her youth clubs and they said they'd buy her a laptop and take her on trips and things but we never heard from them again. There's meant to be support in place but it didn't happen. They did nothing for her.

Some families, it must be said, cope admirably. Many partners, parents and children are compassionate and helpful, and a lot of the patients I speak with are filled with gratitude for their assistance, both practically and psychologically. In a few cases, individuals met and built relationships with partners following their diagnosis. One husband was described by a patient as 'so immensely supportive it's unbelievable. He really is fantastic', and this is not exceptionally uncommon.

Patterns of mistrust

The questions to raise philosophically at this point are manifold. Is it possible to say with any certainty, given the varied and complex axes on which these systems of understanding each other turn, that we are witnessing a pattern here, and a meaningful metaphysical one at that? What makes some people, for want of a better description, 'believe' the fibromyalgia patient in their lives where others are filled with misgivings? Furthermore, isn't an important question not just what how others react to fibromyalgia but what effect this reaction has on the patients themselves?

One approach to these questions is to try to apply some common-sense reasoning. Patients generally report some form of alienation and disaffection from others following their development of fibromyalgia, and the causes of these dissolutions appears remarkably consistent. They appear to be, as I have already outlined, based on a foundational epistemic diminishing of the patient's explanation for their situation, exasperated by the additional effort maintaining social relations now required. In short, it is hard to retain cordial relations with someone who you believe has brought their condition upon themselves or, worse, is fabricating illness in return for material gain, especially if doing so requires more effort on your part to accommodate the new needs of the relationship.

A slightly archaic and little recognised linguistic distinction may come in useful here. In everyday use, there is no difference between 'mistrust' and 'distrust'. That is to say, they are synonyms. However, there is a subtle dictionary distinction between them: to distrust is to be wary on the basis of experience or reasoning, whereas to mistrust is to be generally uneasy on an intuitive basis. We distrust specific people who have a history of lying to us; we mistrust others even if they personally have given us no reason to and we can provide no rationalisation beyond a general feeling of discomfort.

The purpose of drawing a line between these two words is to then use them specifically in relation to fibromyalgia. In general when people encounter individuals with contested illnesses they mistrust them, and if they are closer to the situation then this mistrust may evolve into the more *active* distrust or transform into support and solidarity. Of course what must be kept in mind is that this transition from mistrust to something else is not conducted in a vacuum: what individuals are faced with is not some purely theoretical entity, 'fibromyalgia', but rather the living, breathing flesh of the thing inside the body of a person they may already have reason to dislike or inclination to disbelieve. What is more interesting for me is pursuing the source of the initial *mis*trust, because it suggests that the metaphysical dice are loaded in a particular way.

In order to talk about the effect of this mistrust, I first need to talk about patients and their complicated relationship with the organic or nonorganic nature of their symptoms. Often, sufferers understand these concepts as proxies. So, when others, whether doctors or people around them, question the source of their pain, they take this to mean that they were suggesting it is psychological in origin. This, then, becomes a proxy for two tightly woven strands of resentment: that this means their pain is self-inflicted and that they have control over their symptoms. Furthermore, this also implies a strong degree of agency: the thought that if they so wanted then patients could stop being ill by force of will or by changing something about their person. This overall impression is consistent with Sontag's (1978) observation that illness is often strongly associated with psychological and temperamental inadequacy, particularly in cases where scientific knowledge is limited or ambiguous. Comments from patients like the following were common:

> We don't choose to have this illness, we don't want to be like this, you know we'd do anything really to get better. People spend ridiculous amounts of money just trying to get better, so desperate to be free from the pain.

Nestled in this and similar reactions by patients is the process I outlined immediately above; the implication of choice and the suggestion of a willingness to be ill greeted by patients highlighting the lengths undertaken to be relieved of symptoms as evidence of the absolute and unalterable captivity of their condition.

Analytically, it seems unproblematic to suggest that pain may be emotional in origin but still subconscious and therefore fundamentally out of a person's control. Indeed, this is many a sympathetic doctor's position. The pain is very much real, they say, and there is no doubt that you are feeling the way you say you are, it just happens that in the absence of physical signs we believe the cause to lie elsewhere.

In practice however, many patients, though willing to countenance traumatic experiences as a trigger event and accept stress as a major aggravating factor, maintain an almost unbreakable link between, for want of a better term, psychological origin and being responsible for your symptoms. I say 'for want of a better term' because it does seem as though there should be a distinction drawn between the type of 'psychological origin' patients reject. Surveys show that patients are as likely to cite emotionally painful events in their lives (abuse, breakups, etc.) as they are external physiological causes (viruses for example), but this acceptance of causality is distinct from believing that they are in pain because they are depressed, or because they are suffering ongoing emotional problems (Neerinckx et al., 2000; Häuser et al., 2006; van Wilgen et al., 2008). The point of conception, so to speak, must remain external and in the past even if psychological. A good example of this is the following patient, who agreed with her doctors that overwhelmingly negative psychological incidents in her past had led to her fibromyalgia, but that this previous emotional experience did not mean that her current symptoms were psychological. 'Something happens that just rewires your body,' she told me, 'my body's just wired wrongly now.'

It is worth noting that some patients would agree with the proposition that their symptoms have an entirely emotional base and that there is little physiologically amiss in their bodies. However, they are in a bind, because being apparently cognisant of this aetiology of fibromyalgia does little to change your experience of the disease. As one patient put it in relation to doing an activity, she felt she *knew* she could participate but this knowledge itself would not prevent the pain she experienced during or reduce the soreness and fatigue she suffered afterwards. It is not difficult to see why this kind of epistemic framework is unappealing to most patients.

This problem of distinguishing 'psychological' from physiological is compounded by the phenomenology of the symptoms themselves, which appear to patients to be overwhelmingly biological. A lot of the issues that fibromyalgia patients have are too weird, too disconnected from their brain, too much of a physical hindrance to appear as though they could be psychological to patients. They often seem independent of mood and more affected by biological events (i.e. the pain and flare-ups that patients report after any period of exercise or following a viral infection), and it seems greatly incongruous to individuals that their symptoms are entirely psychological when they live rich emotional lives alongside varying degrees of pain and other problems. Put simply, if your condition is said to be caused by depression or other emotional dysfunction, then how is it possible to have a 'good' week, where you are productive and happy but still suffer from all the symptoms of fibromyalgia? For some, trying to untangle this causal mess starts to feel futile as time wears on. As a patient told me:

> I am now at the stage where I'm not actually all that interested in what caused it, I would just like to know what 'it' is and how I can get better. I am open to the idea that it may be caused by emotional factors but the very real physical symptoms seem inexplicable, unpredictable and totally random.

I think that the strangeness and physicality of the symptoms described above suggests on an intuitive level to patients that what they are feeling in their bodies is separate to their mind, even if it may have been caused as some point in the past by emotional dysfunction. This process also serves to remind us of the causal presumptions we make about disease. As one patient said:

> I can remember working with people that said they had fibromyalgia and I was thinking to myself, yes, well, what emotional problems do you have? Until it happened to me. I think there is definitely an emotional aspect to it but that's definitely not … when my legs cramped up I knew, this is not emotional.

It has been noted for some time that fibromyalgia patients rate their quality of life as lower than healthy controls, individuals with much more 'serious' conditions and doctors' appraisals of their situation based upon clinical evidence (Burckhardt, Clark and Bennett, 1993; Kaplan, Schmidt and Cronan, 2000; Hoffman and Dukes, 2008; Lee et al., 2017). Depending on your perspective, this might suggest a few different things. Firstly, that fibromyalgia patients are depressed exaggerators who have lost touch with the reality of their condition and do not have an appreciation of true hardship within illness. That is to say, they are not happy because *they are not happy*, which is also causing their symptoms. Or, it may point towards an under-appreciation and misunderstanding on the part of doctors and lay individuals as to the restrictive and devastatingly painful core of the disease. Or, to offer one more viewpoint, it may be that the social situation that patients find themselves in restricts their ability to develop 'wellbeing within illness'.[3] In other words, they are unable to adjust to the world around them because it refuses to adjust to

3 'Wellbeing within illness' is a phrase used to describe the idea that though serious sickness is no doubt a difficult experience, it does not necessarily lead to a major reduction in 'wellbeing', or quality of life. That it does in the case of fibromyalgia and other contested diseases contrasts with most other chronic illnesses and traumatic events, where an unpredicted and consistent level of happiness is often self-reported following the initial effects of a negative transformative experience. It is

them. This might also explain the 'exaggeration' of symptoms: when we are not heard, we shout. I do not know why fibromyalgia patients appear less capable of achieving mental peace within their condition than others with chronic illness, but I suspect that the last point raised above plays a role. The psychological burden of being, to put it lightly, misunderstood, and the way in which this specific type of miscommunication (both between yourself and others – the inability to express your pain – and between your own body and your conceptualisations of it) haunts your interactions with the world cannot be conducive to positive mental health.

Organicity and legitimacy

Two main things strike me when thinking about patients and their attitudes towards organicity and legitimacy. The first is the abject poverty of the dualism as it is understood implicitly by most patients at providing a framework for the messages they receive from their body. This is a banal point, and one much explored elsewhere over a number of years in relation to patient experience in medicine generally and in reference to fibromyalgia specifically.[4]

The second is that this could easily be conceptualised as the frequently observed 'stubbornness' of patients in relation to aetiology and organic symptoms, which has often been regarded as an impediment to recovery. The argument goes that in clinging to strictly biological explanations and refusing to consider alternate causal possibilities, patients are harming their chances of getting better because they are not addressing what some see as the 'real' cause of their pain: a deep underlying unhappiness. Furthermore, in pursuing treatment plans based upon false premises, they actively harm their bodies through over-medication and other attempts to alleviate their symptoms such as resting for long periods or turning to untested medicines obtained outside of mainstream medical systems. Over time, this adherence to physical aetiology hardens, becoming part of a fibromyalgia patient's identity, the illness itself becoming a 'way of life' (Ford, 1997, p. 7).

posited that in these cases we overestimate how damaging to our happiness illness will be and underestimate our personal ability to adapt (see Carel, 2016b).

4 For two seminal papers on the role of dualism in medicine, see Sullivan (1986) and Engel (1977). Demitrack (1998, p. 671), for instance, writes about chronic fatigue syndrome and fibromyalgia: 'These characteristics of the two illnesses, namely, profound somatic distress in the absence of any grossly evident biological dysfunction, and their apparent close association with physical and emotional stressors has confounded the traditional, dualistic Western medical model in its attempt to conceptualize them. In a broad sense, these problems serve to frame the basic dilemma for these two conditions: What is their proper place in modern medical thought? Contemporary medical and psychiatric nosologies are most comfortable with unitary illness classifications that demand that an illness be seen fundamentally as either physical or psychological in nature.'

Kroll-Smith and Floyd (1997) have written about this process of seeking biomedical explanations above all else in relation to multiple chemical sensitivity. They label it a 'practical epistemology' whereby patients reconfigure biomedical logic and utilise scientific rhetoric to render their condition comprehensible to themselves and others.[5] They argue that these patients sit at the intersection of modernity and post-modernity, neither giving themselves wholly to a medical system which cannot explain their symptoms physiologically nor privileging their subjective experiences above all else. Propelling this process is an understandable pragmatic desire on the part of patients to make sense of their illnesses through the available and socially powerful tools they find around them.

What is interesting to me is how the pragmatism of identity-building in relation to contested illness is shaped by non-medical factors. The attribution of symptoms to physiological dysfunction despite a lack of substantial evidence is frequently explained in terms of stigma, responsibility, legitimacy and delusion, and it is the exact interactions in which these concepts crystallise that I would like to focus on.

It certainly appears, in reading the literature about fixed illness beliefs and considering Hacking's looping theory, that the points of contact portrayed as most important in establishing this belief system are between institution (or institutional representative) and subject, doctor and patient, the diagnosis and the diagnosed.

In fact, the situation for a number of patients (perhaps all) is more complicated than this. The classic Hacking loop does exist to a degree, insofar as we can trace the development of the fibromyalgia concept through its different diagnostic criteria (i.e. the ACR 1990 criteria followed by the 2010 update), the growth of patient organisations and condition-specific dialect (fibro fog and flare-up), the 'accepted' aetiological model and so on. Indeed, it is certainly true that you can *be* a 'fibromyalgia patient' in a way you couldn't half a century ago.

But what also appears evident is the manner in which this 'identity' is stable but also exists alongside more fractured, antagonistic conflicts over the meaning of fibromyalgia. Conflicts not with doctors or medical classifications, but with people encountered on a day to day, person to person basis. The basic premise of this idea is as follows. In 2019, a fibromyalgia patient may well have a doctor who they are happy with, who is sympathetic, willing to help and genuinely believes they are ill and in need of medical care. They may subscribe to a conceptualisation of their illness such as that promoted by Yunus, which affords them an adequate explanation of what they are feeling

5 An example of this in practice would be the importance placed on scientific 'sounding' diagnoses. See Jason et al. (2002) for a discussion of the implications of different semantic choices in relation to disease names and chronic fatigue syndrome.

in somatic terms (Yunus 1983; Yunus 2011; Yunus 2015). It may be also that they have friends in the patient community with whom they share their experiences and whose companionship allows them to feel comfortable and legitimised in their symptoms. Now, in this scenario, the relationship between patient and category is static and benign, and possesses little of the friction and dynamism we might expect to see in an ordinary interactive kind. However, there remains real tension between categorisation and self-concept, it just occurs outside of these institutional frameworks. It happens in car parks and kitchens.

Because if patients are prone to taking 'psychological origin' as a proxy for a wide range of other, negative inferences, even if this is not what is meant by the doctor who suggests it, then this chain of reasoning could be expected to be prevalent across the population.[6] Which means that in terms of categorical negotiation, fibromyalgia patients find themselves grouped not necessarily by their actual diagnosis, but by where that diagnosis leads: so they are categorised as individuals in control of their symptoms, as malingerers, as emotional unstable and so on. To react to this by doubling down on a categorical definition that centres around physiological dysfunction makes perfect sense, as the inferences from this are the exact opposite: no control of symptoms, understandably emotionally distressed as a result, entitled to both social and financial benefits.

The vital loops then are not between individuals and institutions but between people outside of such structures entirely. To simplify this, it is not just that fibromyalgia patients tend to prefer biological explanations in the clinic, it is that to exist in a society that so quickly makes the leap from 'psychological' to 'accountable' as someone with fibromyalgia becomes unacceptable to our sense of self if we do not postulate an understanding of the disease and of ourselves which promotes an organic base or physiological process over and above emotional factors. This then, is the fallout from the mistrust of which I outlined above: the feeling that others around you encounter your disease in a certain way and the ultimate necessity of proving them wrong so that you can continue to be an individual who has been struck down by circumstance and not by a malignant force of their own making.

Is this process dynamic? A central tenet of Hacking's distinction between interactive kinds and indifferent ones is that the former not only get changed by their categorisation but that this then leads to a change in the way they are categorised. In this way, the category 'wanders'. With fibromyalgia and the interpersonal (rather than institutional) loop I have described above, I would argue that dynamism is in evidence. The attitudes of non-medical persons that patients face, as described in this chapter, pressure them subconsciously

6 Survey data on lay perception of fibromyalgia is lacking, but qualitative reports from patients about their interactions with others in this research and elsewhere would seem to support this statement.

towards particular explanations of their condition and to act in certain ways as a result (whether it be 'wearing a mask' because you don't think others will understand or pestering the doctor for more tests). They also lead the patient to conceptualise not only their condition in a particular way that diminishes stigmatising inferences but also to reconfigure their entire life history.

In turn, the solidifying of illness belief and the alienation felt by patients fuels community action and 'oppositional consciousness', leading to public information campaigns and fundraising activity.[7] One aim of this politicisation of the disease is to increase biomedical research, but another key objective is to affect attitudes, to change the perceptions of those who fibromyalgia patients encountered pejoratively at the beginning of this process.[8]

Thinking back to the first half of the book, I believe that it is by the examination of these interactions that we can make the most sense of Tekin's pursuit of mechanism within Hacking. That is to say, she poses questions about the nature of the selves who are being 'made up', and here I reply that in the case of fibromyalgia a major factor in a patient's 'loop' is the extent to which they can balance their self-concept against the various pressures exerted upon it by their surrounding social environment. Some do this by accepting their (and other's) conceptual ignorance of fibromyalgia, but many are unable to do so, or feel that doing so would delegitimise their pain and leave them at a disadvantage not just in terms of personal validation but also in relation to obtaining the sick role and its attendant benefits.

I asked then: 'How much does the immediate social environment of an individual alter their self-concept?' and I am now in a position to say that this does not lead to glib and obvious truisms, (because I am not framing it in general terms but rather Hacking's parameters); it is instead a question that

7 I have borrowed this term from feminist studies, but I believe it is applicable here (and it is often used in relation to health movements): 'before members of oppressed groups can act collectively, they usually must develop an oppositional consciousness. That is, they must come to see themselves as members of a group, regard their life situations as unjust, find a common interest with other members of the group in opposing that injustice, consider the injustice due to structural inequalities, and believe the injustice can be diminished or ended through their collective actions' (Groch, 2001, p. 65).

8 This attempt to 'change minds' occurs across plenty of other controversial, mostly mental, conditions and is supported by the fact that in some cases legitimising conceptions of illnesses without overwhelming scientific support have 'caught hold' of the public mind (for example the transformation of depression from personal failing into physiochemical imbalance). This is supported by survey data (e.g. Furnham and Telford, 2012). Though some, such as David Healy, would argue that this process is driven largely by pharmaceutical manipulation and agitation (Healy, 2004; Healy, 2012), I would suggest that in contested illnesses (such as the ones discussed in this thesis) this occurs in tandem with patient movements rather than as a dominating factor. Both groups want roughly the same thing – a responsibility absolving, stigma reducing, biomedical explanatory model of disease – though for admittedly very different reasons.

provokes fruitful results upon contemplation. Illness belief is inherently social, and though its negotiation may begin in a medical setting it does not end there. Whatever the trials and tribulations patients have with doctors, these are underlined and in some cases caused by the belief systems about illness reinforced constantly by those around them. The recalibration of the self within illness that fibromyalgia forces upon patients is coordinated in light of their overall social situation, of which medical encounters can play a relatively small part.

A site where this adjustment plays out most dramatically is often in the workplace where, as we will see in the next chapter, work, willingness to work and access to social security act as proxies again for these issues of self. The message is the same as here though, that it is the non-medical encounter that shapes an individual's categorical identity as much as any interactions with medical structures and their representatives, if not more so.

Chapter 9

Work and welfare

Introduction

A strong theme among patients when discussing their condition is a willingness, desire and ability to work that had been curtailed by their illness and compounded both by inflexible workplaces and the impression they receive from others that they are regarded as workshy or trying to game the system. This process often takes place in the shadow of struggles against clunky and rigid bureaucracy to be awarded social security payments on the basis of long term sickness. Despite these issues, many patients do continue to work in some capacity. Often, it is the attitudes of others that formed the greater part of a patient's resentment in relation to work:

- 'It wouldn't occur to me not to work. I'm not sponging off the government getting benefits, I just need a bit of help. I paid into it for twenty years, it's not like I've never done anything.'
- 'There is no way I would have given up my salary by choice and given up a job I enjoyed doing and everything else, you don't just do that.'
- 'I don't want to stay at home and watch daytime television, I want to work.'

Patients frequently make the point that they have always worked, sometimes held multiple jobs at once, and that they were not 'the sort' to try and get something for nothing. Employment brings with it multiple social benefits – regular interactions with others, raised self-esteem, intellectual challenges, status – and many patients regarded it as fundamental to their identity (Henriksson, Liedberg and Gerdle, 2005; Löfgren, Ekholm and Öhman, 2006). It also undoubtably (and perhaps for some most importantly) serves a fiscal purpose. Without work, or with reduced working hours, patients with fibromyalgia find their lives are more restricted financially and their reliance on others increased. Particularly bristling for some is the idea that they should be grateful they no longer have to work, or that they can now work part time:

> I get remarks like 'Oh, you're so lucky working part time', and I think 'Well, I used to bring home two and a half grand a month and now I bring home eight hundred pounds.' That's not lucky, that's not good. I'm doing a job I don't even want to do because it's the only thing I can get with those hours.
>
> I can't tell you how badly I would love to be working outside of the home but it's just not physically possible ... not only do you miss the money that you would be making but you miss the social interactions of speaking with other adults and you know, being out of the four walls of your home. People don't look at it that way, they say 'Oh, she's lucky, she doesn't have to work, she gets to sit at home on her butt.' I don't want to sit at home on my butt!

Work is symbolic for a lot of patients. It stands for their lives pre-illness, but also for evidence of their truthfulness and sincerity. They use their CVs as bulwarks against insinuations and accusations of laziness and scrounging. If they were indeed trying to use sickness as a way of evading employment, then why have they got no history of such evasion? Why, in fact, are their lives often evidence of the opposite: hard work over a number of years, frequently in more than one job at once? Why would they, as many do, have sought flexible working arrangements or work on a part time basis in response to the needs of their condition if their only aim was to avoid work?[1]

Beneath the (understandable) bitterness and anger of these questions lie key aspects of illness and work in western society that fibromyalgia patients collide with: justice and fairness. What frustrates sufferers is the fact that they are not afforded the same allowances as other sick individuals, despite feeling strongly that they are just as ill, and that they have contributed the requisite amount to have earned reparations. This brings to mind the Parsonsian sick role touched upon in the first part of this book, that of an acceptable forfeiting of social responsibilities in case of illness in return for certain actions on the part of the sick individual themselves (i.e. following doctor's orders, trying to get better, etc.).

As Stewart and Sullivan (1982, p. 1397) have argued, the sick role is idealised theoretically around acute conditions which are characterised by 'by definitional and [patient/doctor] role clarity, consensus and harmony'. In chronic conditions like fibromyalgia where the disease is ill-defined and the symptoms inconsistent, the likelihood of recovering quickly and returning to fulfilling their functional role in society is reduced and thus key components

1 These questions touch upon another, older stereotype of patients with conditions such as fibromyalgia and chronic fatigue syndrome: that they are workaholics who have run themselves into the ground. As one patient told me: 'A lot of us have personalities where we are really hard workers and are always busy, you just don't stop.'

of the sick role are compromised.[2] It has also been argued that the longevity of conditions like fibromyalgia undermines the exemption from certain social responsibilities that the sick role provides because this exemption is predicated on a temporary suspension of ordinary duties rather than one conducted on a permanent or semi-permanent basis (Radley, 1994).

The difficulty of accommodating their experiences into the confines of the traditional sick role does not, however, prevent patients from attempting to do so and from feeling frustrated when they find they are unable to. It has been suggested that this is ordinary illness behaviour, as the sick role narrative of restitution is the dominant reaction to disease and few other options are presented to patients as viable or natural responses to falling ill (Robinson, 1990). Therefore, regardless of its applicability to their condition, individuals with fibromyalgia will pursue this course of action.

For many patients, the real tension seems not to be that they have failed to fulfil their end of the bargain (as it were), but rather that they are attempting to benefit from the sick role without being regarded by society as ill at all, or that somehow they are ill in the wrong way. The fact of the matter is they have all received, however belatedly and reluctantly, a diagnosis from a medical professional (otherwise they would not be *fibromyalgia* patients at all), traditionally the key to unlocking the sick role, and yet often they struggle to access its benefits. Clearly, it is not true in any straightforward sense that doctors are the only gatekeepers of the privileges of illness – other factors are in play too.

Partly this can be explained by the favouring of physical symptoms within the sick role, and the sense that only biological dysfunctional or traumatic (in the original sense of the word) injuries are sufficiently amoral to be granted special status.[3] Psychological conditions raise the spectre of personal responsibility and, as we have seen, fibromyalgia sits uncomfortably between the mental and the physical. Research such as Glenton's (2003) has shown that the presumed clear distinction between physical and mental disease has particularly deleterious consequences for individuals trying to access the sick role while suffering from conditions that do not align neatly with either grouping.[4] The words she writes about back pain could easily be adapted to the case of fibromyalgia:

> While the expectations of the sick role are particularly inappropriate for the back pain sufferer, these expectations are still very much present

2 This is a longstanding criticism of Parsons's theory (see Segall, 1976).

3 Grey areas exist (e.g. hangovers), but these are mostly uncontroversial.

4 The visibility and consistency of symptoms are also posited as factors unconducive to success in obtaining sick role status in chronic back pain (Glenton's case study); it is worth noting alongside this that Goffman's description of the stigma of 'character blemishes' – weakness of will, deception, dishonesty, etc. – is applicable here. Patients who find the sick role withheld from them are often motivated further in their pursuit by fear of being falsely categorised and finding themselves on the receiving end of such stigma (see Goffman, 1968).

> among back pain sufferers and their surroundings. Rather than challenge those concepts about sickness and suffering that appear to be tied to the delegitimisation of their experiences, the back pain sufferers … try to fit into the system by striving to live up to the expectations of the sick role.
> (Glenton, 2003, p. 2249)

A further aspect to this problem is the simple observation that diagnoses are not monolithic entities: they come in many shades and while medical legitimacy may inform social legitimacy, it does not do so in a blanket fashion. Stigmatised, underdetermined diagnoses like fibromyalgia lack the credibility of other medical labels. As one patient said: 'fibromyalgia itself as a name has developed quite a stigma because of so many years of being considered a, quote unquote, "trash can diagnosis"'. For conditions like fibromyalgia, the centrality of the doctor/patient relationship to the enactment of legitimisation in the sick role is called into question because being given a stamp of approval (of sorts) by a medical professional is not enough.

Diagnosis is, in the words of Annemarie Jutel (2011, p. 18), 'the *making real* of conceptual categories'. When confronted with a conceptual category as confused, as imprecise, as hologrammatic, as fibromyalgia, it is no surprise that in our attempts to *make it real*, we struggle.

Beyond the diagnosis

A diagnosis offered by a doctor is just one node in a larger network of acceptance. I am talking of the broad bureaucratic structures that surround a patient – their workplace's attitude to illness, the decisions made by social security services and, if under a system like that in the US, the judgement of health insurance companies. All of these are interrelated to some degree, and all work to different parameters of disease. It may well be the case that even though their symptoms are verified by a physician and a diagnosis is proffered, the patient is unable to take time off work because their employers do not recognise their condition or they find themselves without care because their insurance does not cover them (Dumit, 2006).

Inevitably, patients have mixed experiences. Some, like Samuel (who I described earlier), feel they have been forced out of their jobs. Commonly, they find themselves in a bind: their condition makes work harder for them and makes them less appealing to their employers, reducing their workplace capital significantly, often to the point of being made redundant or being removed in some other way (Samuel for instance was forced to leave his job on a technicality after his driving licence was revoked due to his seizures), but their sickness is not taken seriously enough for them to achieve the concessions we might associate with other diseases. Thus their ability to renegotiate their workplace position is severely constrained.

Some patients do secure favourable adjustments in their terms of employment, either by going part-time or reducing their workload. Those that are able to do this are often those who had been working at the same place for a significant amount of time:

> Work are very lenient with me and they have supported me all the way through, but they have seen me from start to finish. They've seen that I have gone from someone who's been healthy, active, jolly, the lot, to someone who sits at her desk now, does as much work as I can before I know I'm going to fall asleep or start lagging or not be able to get done what I need to get done, having regular rest breaks and things like that. So they've seen the transition.

The point could be made that it is the case with nearly all workplace disputes that longevity plays an important role, but what I'm interested in is the specific view of disease presented to employers in the quote above. The patient feels that the salient point here is that her colleagues were witnesses to her transition from health to illness, and that they have therefore alternative evidence to the myriad ambiguities present in fibromyalgia with which to arrive at a judgement. Their sympathy and accommodation is enacted on the basis of the patient's visible transition from one state to another.

These allowances are not afforded to fibromyalgia patients trying to find new employment; without a view of their previous self in the collective minds of their co-workers, they are much more likely to be regarded with suspicion. Observing a patient 'from the beginning' provides those around them with a counterfactual to their illness: it prevents the explanatory void surrounding their symptoms leading necessarily to distrust. In short, seeing a patient transition from one type of person to another, one full of energy to one who is lethargic, provides another form of evidence. Their symptoms may be inconsistent and vague now, but they still represent something significantly removed from how that person was before.

Outside of work, patients can struggle accessing welfare payments (Dumit, 2006). Many, as previous earners and breadwinners, find the process humiliating. A common complaint is that the way in which incapacity is 'tested' (i.e. established as legitimate, does not align with the way that fibromyalgia *is*). Personal assessments based upon ability to do simple tasks and verbal reasoning, as well as unconscious (or perhaps conscious) bias due to the appearance of the patient, do not take into account the inconsistency of fibromyalgia symptoms or the effect exertion has on patients in the medium term:[5]

> Because of the way they word the forms it's very difficult to explain to them that it is not always about what we can do at the time, but how it affects us afterwards. If we were to go and do an eight-hour day when

5 The wholly functional, static assessment procedure employed by government contractors has been criticised on this basis and others (see McCartney, 2012).

> we're on our feet all day, next day we're not going to be able to move. They don't allow for that kind of disability. In their eyes a disability can be seen and it's immediate and if you take painkillers that should be the answer to everything.

Many patients, as any perusal of a fibromyalgia forum will demonstrate, believe that these kinds of assessments are a base form of cynicism, an attempt by government organisations to save money at the expense of patient needs. No doubt too, they feel that the inconsistency of their symptoms and the lack of biomarkers further devalue their diagnosis and give an inch of disbelief to individuals looking to take a mile:[6]

> When I went for a medical, the person that I saw said that I made 'adequate eye-contact'. This person in actual fact did not look at me once during the entire meeting, and I was deemed fit for work.
>
> You are made to feel guilty by the way they do things and they seem to think if they see you walking about outside then you're fine, but they don't see when you get into the house again and collapse into a heap from just walking up the road and back. It's really, really difficult and it is an attitude that they need to change.

These complaints again orbit around ideas of justice and fairness, demonstrated not only by patient's frustration at not receiving some form of compensation (and what might also be termed symbolic acknowledgement) for their condition, but by their anger at others who they believe to unjustly collect state support:

> We've got a girl next door who is twenty-five years old, the government pays for her house because she's got a five-year-old child. She does nothing but lay around the place, sunbathe in the garden and talk on her phone, and it's like, 'Why do I have to go and work and you don't?' You know what I mean? It's madness how someone that's healthy can get that but not someone like me.

Some patients echo these sentiments in a more reflective way, acknowledging the difficulty that fibromyalgia poses to what is a primarily bureaucratic, not medical, framework of administration. They consider the acts of true malingerers to have diminished the credibility of subjective reporting of illness,

6 This is echoed by other studies: 'When the etiology of disease is controversial … or when the existence of a disease is questioned by the medical establishment, as in the case of … fibromyalgia … it becomes difficult to access economic support from workers' compensation systems in the event of disability' (Lippel, 2008, p. 47).

created a more suspicious atmosphere and made it a more difficult process for those who are legitimately sick:

> I think that people who have cheated the system, have claimed when they shouldn't, they've made it harder for the rest of us who are genuinely poorly. I don't know how the system can be changed to make it fairer. Especially as you could be having a particularly bad day, you could be having a middling day, you could be having a good day. That's never taken into account. They just judge you on what they see that day.

Fibromyalgia patients are of course not alone in these frustrations: from the very introduction of social security provision for the sick (whether from the state or through mutual organisations), arguments about legitimate eligibility for assistance have formed the centrepiece of most debates around the just administration of the system and the larger part of complaints against it, both in North America and the UK (Prince, 2008; Macnicol, 2011). In fact, the risk of malingering was highlighted as one of the three main potential pitfalls of introducing National Health Insurance (a forerunner to the NHS) in the first place. Under the current system, recent changes have seen the introduction of the Personal Independence Payment, designed to replace the Employment and Support Allowance and provide individuals with financial support to cover the cost of long-term health conditions. It is not in theory linked to the ability to work or the condition itself but rather the practical effects of a disease or disability on an individual's functional capacity. However, to what extent this idea is enacted in practice remains open to question.

Epistemic tension

The epistemic tension at the heart of these policies is clear: whose assessment of incapacity is to be given the most weight? Whose definition is the most legitimate? For fibromyalgia patients who may have struggled against what they see as the undermining and dismissive attitudes of doctors, the prejudiced and hurtful views of friends and family and potentially financially incapacitating issues with employment, having their disease, or the effects of their disease, questioned on a similar basis in the welfare system may well contribute further to the process of solidification of illness belief I have described above.

Patients are reacting in this case against rigid and false categorisation: the view that if, as some people around them believe, they have agency and control over their condition, then the seeking of welfare payments is a logical step on the path of malingering. In this scenario sufferers therefore have another incentive to emphasise the biomedical aspects of their functional impairment, because it is these components that provide best 'evidence' of their inability to complete tasks and detract from the idea that it is simply one person's word against another. In short, although social security benefits are theoretically assessed functionally in the UK, in practice this translates into a hardening of illness belief on behalf of patients, who feel that an inability to prove the legitimacy of their disability behind its functional effects automatically places them in a highly stigmatised category, that of the benefits 'scrounger' or 'cheat'.[7]

It can also lead to a false public projection of illness. An example from one of the patients I spoke to is illustrative here:

> My partner and his son walked up Ben Nevis a few weeks before I met him and I thought that that, for me, was a pipe dream, to even consider doing that. I printed out a picture of the walk that they did and wrote on it 'you can do this' … Well, in July, we went to Scotland, we went to Ben Nevis and I got a third of the way up. For me this was a phenomenal achievement, something I am immensely proud of. What's really sad from my point of view is that I could not post my pictures on Facebook and say I did this, I got a third of the way up Ben Nevis, I couldn't … I wanted to shout it from the rooftops but I didn't dare because I didn't want to jeopardise my benefits, I didn't want people to judge me differently.

Encapsulated in this story are many of the elements I have been discussing. By hiding her achievements within illness – her capacity to work around functional difficulties – this individual is demonstrating the pressure faced by people with fibromyalgia to present their illness in a way which accords with society's expectations of a *truly ill* person. That is, someone whose symptoms remain consistent in their ability to incapacitate; someone who does not have fun and climb mountains but rather stays in bed and tries to get better; someone who is entitled to state aid because they are desperately, visibly sick, not because they are tired and achey.

What is interesting is the way fibromyalgia is framed differently by patients in different situations: to their doctors, to their friends, to the state and to themselves, and though it may change shape at different sites the intention beneath the framing remains the same.[8] What I mean by this is that though the precise definitions and explanations offered might vary from situation to situation, the underlying emphasis is unchanged: patients wish to be absolved of responsibility for their symptoms and recognition for their distress that

7 This backdrop of pejorative attitudes is longstanding but has been argued to have worsened in recent years. It is particularly related to those who are seen to be unfairly benefiting from the system, e.g. individuals with subjective, unprovable health complaints like fibromyalgia (Baumberg et al., 2012; Jensen and Tyler, 2015).

8 For example, at a work assessment fibromyalgia might be defined by its functional features, in the clinic by its latest symptoms, to friends often by some heuristic or other and to the individual themselves by wholesale changes to their life and their person.

aligns with their pre-existing notions of sickness and justice. That the presentation of their disease does change from clinic to front room illustrates, I think, how individuals frame the messages their body sends them in order to achieve subconscious goals but also allows us to see the degree of 'acceptability' parts of their condition have in different contexts.

This may well appear to be stating the obvious, but what I am trying to convey here is a sense of convergence. That is to say, when we ask questions about a patient's epistemic stance on their illness, it is impossible to reach an answer without considering the many different sites at which that stance is challenged and renegotiated.[9] What is salient here is that a patient is not afforded a binary relationship with the meaning of their illness: it is constantly in need of justification and explanation. The continued clashing of one person's epistemology against another – the totality of *encounters* and the problem of *recognition*, leave a patient with a conception of their disease defined by what it is not. This process gestates in an individual a stronger sense of what they are going through than any conceptualisation provided by medicine and, to bring it back to Hacking's loop, *makes them up* to a greater degree than their relationship with the knowledge produced about them at an institutional level.

9 The use of 'epistemic' and 'epistemology' in this context simply refers to knowledge generation and its outcomes: what does a patient come to know about their condition and how is that knowledge arrived at? What weight is given to equally underdetermined explanations? Which sources of knowledge are privileged? Specifically, why do patients often end up epistemically understanding their condition in biomedical terms, despite evidence to suggest other conceptualisations are more supported? Does this decision say something about the way that the condition is experienced or does it say something about the smithy in which such beliefs are forged? I believe the answer to the last two questions is yes on both counts.

Chapter 10

Care

Introduction

A patient's care, and their interactions with medicine in general, have received a great deal of scholarly interest, and it is a feature of this work that I have tried to focus on and emphasise the non-medical factors that shape the experiences of fibromyalgia patients.[1] As such, I will not provide an exhaustive or in-depth discussion of the ways in which diagnosis and interactions with doctors affect patients, providing instead a brief overview.

Diagnosis

Much work has been done to establish a 'sociology of diagnosis' (Blaxter, 1978; Brown, 1990; Jutel, 2009; Jutel, 2015), where focus is given to diagnosis as a primary site of transformation for the patient. What is meant by this varies: it could relate to the legal and political functions a diagnosis performs, the psychological shift it may enact, the legitimacy it may confer, or some other way in which receiving a label marks the shift by which a 'contestable subjective state … achieves a more authoritative objectivity' (Madden and Sim, 2016, p. 89).

A diagnosis is not a fleshy thing – it does not exist ontologically. It is a conceptual category that binds the 'biological, the technological, the social, the political and the lived' (Jutel, 2009, p. 294). However, for patients, it is important an immensely real way, performing an informative and therapeutic function, as well as often transmitting to the patient an entirely new *identity* (Jutel, 2011, p. 25). In cases of contested illness, there is a tension to be found in the diagnostic encounter that is not often present in other conditions: the diagnosis itself is lacking in detail and authority, and there is ambivalence (as discussed previously) among some doctors as to the benefits of conveying one

1 For a range of perspectives over time on the doctor–patient relationship in relation to fibromyalgia and other contested illnesses, see Hanh et al. (1994), Åsbring and Närvänen (2002), Werner and Malterud (2003), Dobkin et al. (2003), Wasan et al. (2005), Hayes et al. (2010) and Clark et al. (2013).

at all. Alongside this, there is a resistance to epistemic contributions by the patients themselves, who have either researched their symptoms and offered suggestions or otherwise arrived at the clinic having self-diagnosed. This being said, there is no doubt too that the proffering of a name frequently allays severe concerns that may have developed in patients as to the veracity of their experiences, and the degree to which they trust their experience of their own body (Kralik, Brown and Koch, 2001).

Commonly, in the case of fibromyalgia, the diagnostic process goes as follows: a patient starts suffering fatigue and joint pain, sometimes in a specific place such as the lower back or shoulder. These symptoms continue and do not respond to painkillers while a multitude of tests are conducted and a variety of specialists employed to rule out other, more easily established conditions. Eventually, usually following a referral to a neurologist, physiotherapist or rheumatologist, and perhaps after the administration of a pressure point examination, a diagnosis of fibromyalgia is offered.

A patient told me, for instance: 'Originally we were concerned about MS, did the tests for that, couldn't find anything. Did the tests for everything else, couldn't find anything so we ended up at fibromyalgia.' Others are explicitly aware that theirs is a diagnosis of exclusion:

> Some didn't believe it, said it's all in your head. The rheumatologist I saw just said he didn't think it was a real disease and so what did we expect him to do about it? It isn't anything else that you've got so we might as well call it that but there's nothing I can do.

Some are diagnosed by non-medical professionals to begin with:

> As bad as it sounds, my hairdresser actually identified it. And said 'I really think you might have fibromyalgia,' and I went to the GP and discussed it. So she sent me to the neurologist and she said, 'Oh, I agree. What do you want me to do about it?' Literally in those words. And that was it. But at least I've got a name now and I can understand it a bit better and find more out about it. So even though I did feel as though I'd been treated very flippantly by the neurologist, they did help me put a name to my illness.

These quotes speak volumes about the fibromyalgia patient experience in relation to diagnosis. Often arrived at tangentially and without firm conviction, it nonetheless does offer to many patients a small degree of hope and a semblance of clarity. They have a label and a way of understanding and explaining their symptoms. However problematic this may be, it is for most patients a step up from the uncertainty and alienation of having no name at all for their distress.

Some patients do dispute their diagnosis, conscious of the methodological problems in identifying fibromyalgia. Most of all, they are not satisfied that everything that could have been done had been to locate some other, more biomedical but also, crucially, more *curable* condition. Some patients also feel as though they are on the wrong side of a bureaucratic cost benefit analysis, one that leaves them powerless and under-treated:

> It's almost like it's convenient for them to diagnose it as there's no legal comeback, because I can't sue them, they don't care … You rely on family and friends and your own private money on tests with the hope that something might come up, that they might find something they haven't tested for, that they might have the cure. What if I haven't got fibromyalgia? What if it's something else? I don't know, another rare disease that may be curable or treatable? The best hope for me is that it's not fibromyalgia. But they're not giving me the option because they're not doing enough tests.

This patient's view illustrates the consumer model of patient/doctor interactions in a novel way: here the patient is acting like a consumer, rejecting the judgment of the doctor and demanding a different course of action, but their 'rights' as they see them (to undergo more tests) are being undermined by doctors who still weald the power supposedly stripped from them by precisely this kind of 'consumer' behaviour.

Other patients more faithfully enact the 'doctor shopper' model, switching between professionals until they find one they are happy with.[2] Unlike the sufferer described immediately above, however, the issues patients have with 'bad' doctors revolve in large part around the *manner* of the professional, rather than solely the substance of what they had to say. Patients seek doctors who they feel believe them and are willing to try different therapies, even if they were ignorant or acknowledged themselves that medicine could not offer an entirely cogent explanation or treatment plan. For example, let us look at the experience of the following patient:

> I have no fear of changing doctors if I have one that I don't feel is making sense or listening. I've had orthopaedic doctors that don't even listen, they talk over me and wanted to ignore the pain I'm feeling and pretend it's not there instead of actually looking into it. I've had one that has left me in tears because he was so rude. I was standing there in massive amounts of pain, my shoulder's hurting and yet he's grabbing it and twisting it in all directions, making me scream and telling me there's nothing wrong with it. Obviously I didn't return to him.

2 It should be noted that the concept of 'doctor shopping' can be defined in numerous ways and there is no one universally agreed upon description (Sansone and Sansone, 2012).

What is important to her relationship with her doctor is the respect with which her and her symptoms are treated. Being talked over and having her pain ignored or minimised does more to sour her relationship with a doctor than the ambiguities present in her condition. This is an example of epistemic injustice: the epistemic status of the patient has been minimised and as a result she has been made to feel as if her testimony is ignored because other epistemic sources are given more credence.

Another example can be seen in the following: 'They sent me to another doctor and used the term "women like me" or something. It was a very derogatory statement they had made implying it was all in my mind, kinda hypochondria.'

Fibromyalgia patients often complain that doctors are too quick to reach for a purely psychological explanation which, as we have seen, is somewhat unpalatable for them. There is a distinction to be drawn here, however: believing in the psychological origins of symptoms is separate from believing the symptoms themselves to *be* psychological. To many patients, it makes sense that emotional trauma might cause pain, but it does not follow that the pain itself is anything other than a physiological phenomenon. This gets doubly complicated when we factor in one of the most common comorbidities of the fibromyalgia patient – depression – and the conflicting inferences of doctor and patient, the former often believing the depression to drive the pain and fatigue, the latter certain that the pain they are in is causing them to feel low:

> I know I'm not depressed but when I get an attack of all sorts of different types of pain, when I get an attack of one of those, it sends me into, well, I want to die, I feel suicidal, there's no point in living, I can't go on like this but then I would wake up in the morning and feel better and ready to get on with my day again. So it causes depression … I think my depression was caused by the pain.

It is not necessarily fair to paint the doctor–patient relationship as a wholly antagonistic one in the case of fibromyalgia, though that is often the impression given in the literature (Bieber et al., 2006; Matthias and Bair, 2010; Briones-Vozmediano et al., 2013). Many patients have positive interactions with doctors, forming relationships that are trusting, palliative and just about as good as could be expected given the circumstances:

> I've started with a new doctor. They will do home visits and so far they've been very good. If I make suggestions then usually they are willing to listen. I don't know if it's my background with the nursing or not but they seem to be quite obliging in that way. But it's really difficult to treat this illness.

However, the uncertainties and amorphous definitions that permeate other aspects of fibromyalgia are just as present in the clinic. Being diagnosed is just one step of many towards constructing a meaningful definition of their condition and assimilating it into their present and past experiences. Even a doctor who listens to and trusts the patient may not be able to offer them much in terms of understanding what fibromyalgia 'is':

> It is a relief [to be diagnosed], but unfortunately you sit down and go, well I've been diagnosed, now what? They don't actually tell you anything when you are diagnosed, they're not helpful at all.
>
> The rheumatologist did all the tests for arthritis and stuff and then said, I don't like giving this diagnosis, it makes me anxious in case I've missed something but I think it's fibromyalgia. And he didn't know anything about it. He kinda said there's not much to tell, there's not much I can do about it and that was it.

The lack of information provided to patients, underlined by genuine clinical uncertainty, makes narrative construction more difficult. Patients look elsewhere to construct their meaning of fibromyalgia, since that offered by healthcare professionals is so devoid of detail. This, combined with the impotence of the treatment plans, drive individuals to learn more about their condition from a wide range of sources. Filtering of information is necessary to avoid absorbing false information or being exploited but often patients feel like they have nothing to lose by trying something new:

> You do tend to go online because you're just desperate to find out things. I'm very aware that there's a lot online, particularly from America, where people will offer a cure for it, they write books called *A Cure for Fibromyalgia* … Well of course there's no cure at the moment. You've got to sift it in your own mind and take out the relevant bits.
>
> When you're diagnosed with something and the doctor can't help you, you do get a little desperate looking for things, and when you see what people are offering in the way of pills and potions and this cream and that cream and all the rest of it, and the prices they are charging, and they're not necessarily going to do anything anyway. But of course people do get very desperate when they're in pain and fatigue and all the rest of it. You do tend to go for things.

The bottom line is, I think, that many patients would agree with one individual I spoke with, who told me that when she was diagnosed: 'I didn't have a clue what it was'. The patients I talked with who were involved in community support groups indicated to me that it was common for a sufferer to know next to nothing about their condition when they were diagnosed. What they learnt about it they discovered through their own research and their interactions with other patients, which aligns with the idea that key to the construction of meaning in this situation is the non-medical world of the patient, or perhaps more accurately their non-medically mediated world.

In the search for a mechanism behind the cultural transmission of symptoms highlighted by Shorter and Showalter, I find little to support their arguments. Patients are frequently ill long before they were diagnosed and construct most of what they come to know about their condition following a long period of uncertainty. No doubt framing of symptoms in light of information later learned occurs, but to say that these problems are shaped entirely and always by culture does not appear to me to be accurate.[3]

Furthermore, the centrality of the doctor–patient relationship to the production of specific symptom types, as described by Shorter, is not evident and neither are media exposure (at least on the face of it) or shifting medical paradigms major factors. The symptoms experienced by patients in most cases appear to predate their meaningful assimilation of them into any kind of conceptual framework by quite a long time – decades in some instances – and doctors, as discussed above, are often able to offer patients little in the way of explanation or information about fibromyalgia, or are actively reluctant to do so, suggesting a diminished element of iatrogenicity, if there is any present at all.

A lack of intertextuality

Showalter argues for intertextuality as a means of understanding how similar symptoms appear to clot around a particular psychosomatic disease. The sum total of reporting and consumption of media surrounding a condition creates for troubled individuals ways in which to be ill – it gives them stories with which to understand what is happening to them and this subconscious interpretation causes symptoms to crystallise in a particular way. This then feeds back into the narrative: if another person feels exactly like this, then there must be some common, base cause.

Although there is an elegance to this idea, and like any other bibliophile I am enamoured by the thought of stories being so *powerful*, when it comes to fibromyalgia patients I do not see narrative as having a formative role. Patients rarely seem to mention news reports, television shows, or other media in the recounting of their illness, and if the intense intertextuality and profound media influence suggested by Shorter and Showalter exists, then its reach is hidden from me. As stated above, most patients appear to live a life in limbo before they are given a diagnosis, and many speak of the ambiguity of information available and the sense of living in a vacuum of information.

3 That is to say, there seems to be a thick heart to fibromyalgia which is independent of or extremely obscurely related to the culture of the patient. Tracing lines between the individual, their symptoms and the culture they are part of is, however, of great difficulty.

What appears more likely to have an impact on their ideas about their condition was their interactions with other patients following diagnosis.

None of this is to say that patients don't tell stories about themselves to make sense of their lives, or that they don't recognise themselves in the stories of others.[4] It is just to point out that this was never the contention, and to say that aligning your experiences within a narrative framework *actively* sought following a diagnosis is significantly different from a state of affairs whereby symptoms start to exist because they are read about, where a patient becomes something to see because they feel seen.

Patient groups

I have included patient support groups in this chapter instead of Chapter 8 because as I worked on this book I began to see more and more that the patient 'community' was not so much something an individual with fibromyalgia automatically joins, but rather a loose network that could be utilised or rejected as they saw fit.[5] In other words, it is more piecemeal than unitary. Almost all patients encounter others with their condition following their diagnosis, whether through joining a group or more passively, and the value of such encounters is inevitably varied. Clearly, a certain amount of commonality and relief can be found from talking to others in the same situation as yourself, but equally patients can have negative experiences, finding patient groups overly pessimistic and defeatist, more focused on bad-mouthing doctors and repeating tales of woe than offering support.

If we start with some of the positives, I would say that these groups – who meet locally, organise events and are largely self-organised – play a particularly important role when a patient has just received their diagnosis and is uncertain about how to proceed. One patient, who runs a support group herself, said:

> It is about giving people the support, including myself really, that you won't get from anywhere else, because only people with the condition can understand how somebody feels. So especially for people when they're newly diagnosed and they're really confused and there's nobody else to turn to and they don't understand it, their families certainly don't understand it, at that point it's nice to be able to talk about it and learn a bit more about it with people who really know.

4 Barker (2005) has detailed the profundity patients attach to 'recognising' themselves in patient literature.

5 By 'patient community' I mean: large organisations like Fibromyalgia Action UK, local support groups, online groups such as patient forums and pages on social media and helplines for those with the disease.

Another said:

> Every new person that comes, they all say they're still alone and no one believes them, and that no one else understands how they feel and they feel like they're the only ones and they don't know how to explain it to their family. That's the general pattern of things when new people arrive.

These quotes touch upon a point that I often hear made, which is that no matter the level of support and sympathy they received from those around them, it is a relief for patients to talk to others with fibromyalgia for the simple reason that they could truly understand what they were going through. This brings to mind the earlier discussion about empathising with another's pain: I would suggest that fibromyalgia patients themselves think that there is something unique, something *other* about the symptoms they experience. What is uncertain is whether this is an intrinsic 'fact' of the condition or whether they arrive at this opinion following repeated interactions with people who never seem to understand the way that they feel inside of themselves.

Some of the patients I have spoken with find that using support groups, in real life or online, calms their anxieties about particular symptoms, especially those on the stranger side. In this immensely connected world, it is not that difficult to find another person who has had or is claiming to have had similar experiences to you, and that can come as a relief:

> I had this weird episode where I, this sounds really bizarre, if I tasted any food or drink, my taste buds, saliva glands or whatever, would just go berserk and so I was on the forum saying 'I know this is bizarre, but has anyone experienced this?' and someone had and they didn't know what it was. And so to go on there and get reassurance that you're not the only one to have these weird and wonderful symptoms, that's reassuring.
>
> So many of the things that people talk about, I go 'Oh my God, me too, it's not just me!' So I feel an acceptance and an understanding in those groups that I don't have a lot of in my real life.

A question that this type of comment raises in my head is: do the negative outcomes of this process outweigh the positives for patients? That is to say, yes patients are able to find others who feel the same as them and feel less alienated as a result, but would they been better off if they had tried to ignore the symptoms entirely rather than fixating (in a loose sense) upon them, putting them into words, talking to others about them, etc.? Certainly, strange symptoms become a lot easier to assimilate into 'the disease' once it becomes evident that other people with fibromyalgia also have the same complaints. And once odd experiences become normalised as symptoms, would it not be understandable if patients began to understand every out-of-the-ordinary experience they had as a fibromyalgia symptom?

Or, to take another tack: does this kind of comment provide a counterbalance to ideas about intertextuality? Patients in the situations above clearly had no precedent for their experiences – no prototype, no story – and it was only through talking with others that they realised they were not the only ones who felt this way. Evidence like this appears to me to make the case that these patients are undergoing something fundamentally similar, even if bizarre.

By asking these questions we can appreciate the complicated ways that communication between patients might interact with their experiences of their body and in turn, through some obscure, little understood mechanism, actually *change* those experiences.

One further function of the fibromyalgia community that patients sometimes find helpful is the sharing of ideas in relation to treatment. A lot of individuals are adverse to the drug-heavy regimes suggested by their doctors and preferred to discuss with other patients what it was that had worked for them, whether that involved a change in diet, a particular type of exercise or meditation. Pooling ideas and success stories locally and online allows patients to feel as though they are in a reciprocal relationship with each other, working together to better manage their symptoms.

However, some patients think that, though they have their place, online forums and local support groups can leave them feeling worse than before: 'One girl I know went to a group but she came out of there feeling so depressed, it was so miserable, not uplifting in any form and she won't be going back. That's what you don't need.' Another patient reported: 'There's a lot of doom and gloom on there [the forums], and I think, "Oh, I can't be dealing with this today", and I don't log on.'

Some of those with fibromyalgia also feel that the ultimate outcome of these group settings – which revolve around discussions of symptoms, experiences with doctors and general tales of problems faced – was a worsening state of health. For them, the mental attitude you take as a sufferer towards your illness is critical:

> I joined different things. It was negative, negative, negative. To the point where I was thinking 'Good God, do something about it! Don't just sit there and whine that you're in bed.' To be in bed all day is not an option. To me, if you lay in bed all day you're making it worse because you're not moving.

Attitudes like this encapsulate for me more than anything my feeling that beneath all the symbolic explanations and oblique theories of medico-cultural interplay, there is a strong element of fibromyalgia and similar conditions that simply *is*. Often, patients possess no knowledge about fibromyalgia before their diagnosis and remain open-minded following it. They try to exercise and eat well, and attempt to maintain a healthy and positive mental attitude. Their experiences with doctors, while not without acrimony, often lead to a mutual and beneficial relationship. They go online and to other patients in search of information and treatment ideas, but do so with a sceptical mind. In other words, as far as I can see, they frequency display little of the characteristic stubbornness or unreasonable behaviour that one might expect to see having read portions of the literature. And through it all they continued to be in pain.

Furthermore, it seems to me that some sufferers define themselves not just against the impressions of others, be it doctors, family or whomever, but also against what they perceive as the 'wrong' attitude towards having fibromyalgia. They do not want to give in to invalidism and are frustrated by those who they thought of as doing so. As one patient said:

> I know that some in my group are perceived as not trying. They think 'Oh, I can't do that so I won't work, I can't do that so I won't do anything.' And it's like, you know, 'You could do a little bit, I'm sure a call centre or something. You could answer the phone.' And some will say 'No I can't do it, I can't do anything.' You have got to try, you have got to push a little bit.

This additional level of interplay – between patients themselves, adds further complexity to the idea that our beliefs about illness are tied up strongly in that against which we define ourselves. I sense that some patients disbelieve others, in precisely the same way that they are disbelieved. I also sense that some patients are irritated by others for giving the condition a 'bad name', for being what appears to be self-involved hypochondriacs, always focusing on the negative. And, to some degree, I believe that within any group of people some will be annoyed by others – shared patient-hood or not. It is always hard to unpick the strands.

Conclusion

My hope is that the materials presented in this book have relayed above all the pure complexity of the issue at hand, and generally point towards the same truism: there is more than one way to skin a cat, just as there is more than one way to become a patient with a contested illness and more than one way to *be* one. I have covered a lot of ground, dipping my toe as I went in various bodies of literature from a range of fields, and my desire is that the resulting analysis has been a holistic examination rather than a superficial and slipshod treatment of a difficult and sensitive topic.

At the beginning of this work, I stated that my aim was:

> … to look in detail at the philosophical context that frames the way contested illnesses are experienced and understood by patients in the early 21st century … The focus of this research is therefore to trace with greater accuracy, and more importantly greater reference to lived experience, the contours of belief and assumption which provide us with our collective map of disease.

I believe that I have succeeded in this aim. Throughout the foregoing chapters I have introduced and discussed a number of ideas which I believe help us to understand the way in which contested illness and, in particular, fibromyalgia patients relate to their condition and, furthermore, elucidate a general sense of our collective idea of disease, as nebulous as that may be. I have also identified and analysed those ideas which I believe to be unhelpful or distracting – ideas such as the notion that philosophers of medicine should focus on the definition of disease problem. Though I offered arguments against this in Chapter 3, let us briefly consider them again in light of the second half of the book.

What, for instance, can the definition of disease literature tell us about fibromyalgia? That it either is or is not a disease, depending on whose schema you employ.[1] This does not resolve any controversies or offer any insight into

1 Naturalists would probably conclude that it is not, normativists that it is. Neither discuss such cases specifically.

the experiences patients have. It remains, in my view, a conceptual distraction. I think that what we can see that in relation to disease we have very often been asking the wrong questions.

Instead of asking *what*, we should be asking *who, how, why* and *at what location*? Diseases are 'defined' constantly, most often by individuals whose definitions carry with them more consequences than those of philosophers. Truly descriptive studies of disease definition will have to give up on the false promise of universality, abandoning this edifice for work which is specific and grounded in examples. We should therefore be looking at how *diseases* are defined, not disease.

Clearly there is a huge medical component to the focus of this work, but what I have emphasised in this book is the extent to which non-medical factors come to bear upon patients. This is true too in relation to disease definition, for much of the literature takes it for granted that in most cases an adequate characterisation of a condition can be found (these form most of the counterexamples) without questioning either the epistemic authority on which that definition is based or asking about the diversity of opinion that may exist among the 'definers'. Disease definition is taken to be a straightforward process enacted by a homogenous group, the philosopher's job being to create a category which captures all of this group's outputs. I hope that in this volume I have shown this method to be based on false premises.

Throughout this work I have also tried to demonstrate the usefulness of collapsing the categories of 'disease', 'illness' and 'sickness'. The epistemic privileging of 'disease' within this schema, despite its original aims at liberation, compound issues that patients face.[2] Treating them as one and the same allows us too to switch more easily between the medical and non-medical encounter, examining all aspects of the way the disease operates rather than trying to delineate different sections of it for piecemeal analysis. We can thus talk about fibromyalgia in terms of pain receptors and welfare payments and self-doubt, because they are all bees of the same hive.

At present the overt link between 'disease' and biomedical signifiers leaves patients shut out of the category and placed in another. Sociologically we say that fibromyalgia sufferers have 'illness' but not 'disease'; for the patients themselves this distinction means they are caught in a netherworld where they feel diseased but are treated as if they are not. A continued recognition and focus on the fact that distinguishing between disease as biomedically defined and sickness as experienced creates a whole category of discontented and dysfunctional patients with little to guide their experience is necessary to understand the problems of these individuals and to make their lives easier.

This work has also, I believe, demonstrated the truth behind the idea that illness presents a unique opportunity to think about our world, our beliefs and ourselves. In other words, disease is ideal philosophical fodder. The

2 A position I share with Annemarie Mol (2003).

breadth and range of topics touched upon in the above discussion pay testament to this notion, and I remain convinced that there are few other topics which so aggressively force the intersection of thoughts about embodiment, mortality, causality, communication and biology. Such cases as I have discussed remain fundamentally unsolved and obscure but they are also insightful and revealing. They make us look twice, they make us consider alternatives.

The opportunities for this kind of philosophising are vast. In this book, I have, for instance, paid particular attention to questions of interiority and trust – both trust in others and confidence about our own bodies. Different gradations of pain, for example, make us question simplistic, unitary models of empathy. If pain comes in different flavours, and I think we can confidently say – biologically and phenomenologically – that it does, then what effect does this have on our ability to appraise pain? To situate it interpersonally and socially? What drives our allocation of empathy? Is it some form of solution aversion, whereby subjective pain complaints act as proxies for anxiety about justice and fair distribution of resources? Or is the presentation of pain, in all its variations, ultimately more important to engendering understanding in others than anything a person might verbally express about the way they feel inside? Though pain is sometimes positioned as the archetypical 'unknowable', I have shown that some forms of pain are treated differently precisely on the basis of which they appear 'known', picked up by medical instruments, allayed by treatment, etched on the faces of patients in a familiar way.

And then come the questions of identity-building, of weighing up the immediacy of physical signals against the social backdrop that gives our experiences meaning, the endless back and forth of categorisation, self-determination and a desire to be comfortable with ourselves physically and psychologically. Individuals with contested illnesses are placed in an impossible bind, for even those among them who are 'model' patients, who hand themselves over fully and acquiescently to medicine, remain in a situation of painful indeterminacy as regards their symptoms and bodies, a state that allows for little development of internal, narrative explanations. It is hard, if not impossible, for patients to live comfortably in a state of *not knowing*, especially given the multitude of pressures that are brought to bear upon them through the inter-personal and bureaucratic encounters that repeatedly ask them to describe, explain and justify that which simply, currently, cannot be.

So what is my conclusion? That it is important to think about illness from all angles, not just medical ones. That the prevailing notion of disease held loosely across the population – more so, in fact across the lay population than the expert – is reductionist, mechanistic, specific; concerned with restitution; hierarchical and deferential to medical expertise in its classification; suspicious of intent and subjectivity; constructed around consistent and visual symptoms, both in the everyday and clinical senses. Individuals encountering disease have a set of preconceptions about it, and as I have detailed, a set of causal expectations. When these expectations are not met, when we do not recognise disease in an individual, then other inferences start to occupy the territory ordinarily reserved for sympathy and assistance. This mode of thinking is reflected not only in the attitudes of lay people but also in how patients experience, rationalise and narrativise their condition. At different sites it is refracted to accommodate various aims – whether in relation to a productive, efficient workforce or a welfare system geared towards saving costs – but retains the same central features. Belief and empathy are fickle, and rely upon the support of a causal matrix; simply communicating distress in an explanatory void is not enough to entitle the patient to what they feel as though they deserve. My conclusion is that the strictures of biomedical thinking are precisely that – a narrowing of vision, a tightening of the imagination. Much in the same way as blinkers prevent horses from being spooked or distracted, our modes of thinking about illness bring clear benefits, but they also act as restraints on the types of information to be considered and the credence we give to it. It becomes incredibly difficult to look at something from a different angle once you have become accustomed to seeing it in a certain way, because such a recalibration comes to require a wholesale adjustment of your viewpoint.

The famous French surgeon Leriche is said to have commented that health is life lived in the silence of the organs. Fibromyalgia patients find their bodies speaking at a frequency we cannot hear. We mistake this for silence, and therein lies the problem.

Bibliography

Aaron, L. A. and Buchwald, D. 2001, 'A review of the evidence for overlap among unexplained clinical conditions', *The Annals of Internal Medicine*, 134, pp. 868–881.

Aaron, L. A. *et al.* 2001, 'Comorbid conditions in chronic fatigue: a co-twin control study', *The Journal of General Internal Medicine*, 16(1), pp. 24–31.

Ahmad, K. and Ramsay, B. 2009, 'Delusional parasitosis: lessons learnt', *Acta Dermato-Venereologica*, 89, pp. 165–168.

Aho, J. A. and Aho, K. 2008, *Body Matters: A Phenomenology of Sickness, Disease, and Illness*, Lexington Books, USA.

Album, D. and Westin, S. 2008, 'Do diseases have a prestige hierarchy? A survey among physicians and medical students', *Social Sciences and Medicine*, 66(1), pp. 182–188.

Alzabin, S. and Venables, P. J. 2012, 'Etiology of autoimmune disease: past, present and future', *Expert Review of Clinical Immunology*, 8(2), pp. 111–113.

Ambrose, K. R., Gracely, R. H. and Glass, J. M. 2012, 'Fibromyalgia dyscognition: concepts and issues', *Reumatismo*, 64(4), pp. 206–215.

Andorno, R. 2007, 'Global bioethics at UNESCO: in defence of the Universal Declaration on Bioethics and Human Rights', in *The Journal of Medical Ethics*, 33 (3), pp. 150–154.

Appignanesi, L. 2009, *Mad, Bad and Sad: A History of Women and the Mind Doctors from 1800 to the Present*, Viarago, UK.

Arnold, L. M. *et al.* 2008, 'Patient perspectives on the impact of fibromyalgia', *Patient Education and Counselling*, 73(1), pp. 114–120.

Arnold, L. M., Hudson, J. L., Keck, P. E., Auchenbach, M. B., Javaras, K. N. and Hess, E. V. 2006, 'Comorbidity of fibromyalgia and psychiatric disorders', *The Journal of Clinical Psychiatry*, 67(8), pp. 1219–1225.

Åsbring, P. and Närvänen, A. L. 2002, 'Women's experiences of stigma in relation to chronic fatigue syndrome and fibromyalgia', *Qualitative Health Research*, 12(2), pp. 148–160.

Åsbring, P. and Närvänen, A. 2003, 'Ideal versus reality: physicians perspectives on patients with chronic fatigue syndrome (CFS) and fibromyalgia', *Social Science and Medicine*, 57(4), pp. 711–720.

Bak, R. *et al.* 2008, 'A review of delusions of parasitosis, part 1: presentation and diagnosis', *Cutis*, 82(2), pp. 123–130.

Barker, K. K. 2005, *The Fibromyalgia Story*, Temple University Press, USA.

Barsky, A. J. and Borus, J. F. 1999, 'Functional somatic syndromes', *Annals of Internal Medicine*, 130, pp. 910–921.

Bartels, E. M. 2009, 'Fibromyalgia, diagnosis and prevalence: are gender differences explainable?', *Ugeskrift for Læger*, 171(49), pp. 3588–3592.

Bass, C. and Halligan, P. 2014, 'Factitious disorders and malingering: challenges for clinical assessment and management', *The Lancet*, 383(9926), pp. 1422–1432.

Baumberg, B., Bell, K. and Gaffney, D. 2012, 'Benefits stigma in Britain', project report for Elizabeth Finn Care.

Bayliss, R. I. S. 1984, 'The deceivers', *The British Medical Journal*, 288(6417), pp. 583–584.

Bellamy, R. 1997, 'Compensation neurosis: financial reward for illness as nocebo', *Clinical Orthopaedics and Related Research*, 336, pp. 94–106.

Bellato, E. *et al.* 2012, 'Fibromyalgia syndrome: etiology, pathogenesis, diagnosis, and treatment', *Pain Research and Treatment*, 2012, article 426130.

Bellow, S. 1975, *Humboldt's Gift*, Vintage, USA.

Betti, V. and Aglioti, S. M. 2016, 'Dynamic construction of the neural networks underpinning empathy for pain', *Neuroscience and Biobehavioral Reviews*, 63, pp. 191–206.

Bieber, C., Muller, K. G., Blumenstiel, K. *et al.* 2006, 'Long-term effects of a shared decision-making intervention on physician-patient interaction and outcome in fibromyalgia: A qualitative and quantitative 1 year follow-up of a randomized controlled trial', *Patient Education and Counselling*, 63, pp. 357–366.

Binder, L. M. and Campbell, K. A. 2004, 'Medically unexplained symptoms and neuropsychological assessment',*The Journal of Clinical and Experimental Neuropsychology*, 26(3), pp. 369–392.

Bishop, J. P. 2011, *The Anticipatory Corpse: Medicine, Power and the Care of the Dying*, University of Notre Dame Press, USA.

Blaxter, M. 1978, 'Diagnosis as category and process: the case of alcoholism', *Social Science and Medicine*, 12, pp. 9–17.

Blease, C., Carel, H. and Geraghty, K. 'Epistemic injustice in healthcare encounters: evidence from chronic fatigue syndrome', *The Journal of Medical Ethics*, 2016, 43 (8), doi:10.1136/medethics-2016-103691.

BMJ, 2002, 'What do you think is a non-disease?', *The British Medical Journal*, 324, p. 7334.

Bolton, D. 2007, 'The usefulness of Wakefield's definition for the diagnostic manuals', *World Psychiatry*, 6(3), pp. 164–165.

Boon, N. A., Colledge, N. R., Walker, B. R. and Hunter, J. A. A. 2006, *Davidson's Principles and Practice of Medicine*, 20th edition, Churchill Livingstone, UK.

Boorse, C. 1975, 'On the distinction between disease and illness', *Philosophy and Public Affairs*, 5, pp. 49–68.

Boorse, C. 1977, 'Health as a theoretical concept', *Philosophy of Science*, 44, pp. 542–573.

Boorse, C. 1997, 'A rebuttal on health', in J. M. Humber and R. F. Almeder (eds), *What is Disease?*, Humana Press, USA.

Boorse, C. 2014, 'A second rebuttal on health', *The Journal of Medicine and Philosophy*, 39(6), pp. 683–724.

Bossema, E. R. *et al.* 2013, 'Influence of weather on daily symptoms of pain and fatigue in female patients with fibromyalgia: a multilevel regression analysis', *Arthritis Care and Research*, 65(7), pp. 1019–1025.

Boulet, L. and Boulay, M. 2011, 'Asthma-related comorbidities', *Expert Review of Respiratory Medicine*, 5(3), pp. 377–393.

Boyd, K. M. 2000, 'Disease, illness, sickness, health, healing and wholeness: exploring some elusive concepts', *Medical Humanities*, 26, pp. 9–17.

Branco, J. C. *et al.* 2010, 'Prevalence of fibromyalgia: a survey in five European countries', *Seminars in Arthritis and Rheumatism*, 39(6), pp. 448–453.

Briones-Vozmediano, E., Vives-Cases, C., Ronda-Pérez, E. and Gil-González, D. 2013, 'Patients' and professionals' views on managing fibromyalgia', *Pain Research and Management*, 18(1), pp. 19–24.

Brown, P. 1990, 'The name game: toward a sociology of diagnosis', *The Journal of Mind and Behaviour*, 11(3–4), pp. 385–406.

Brown, C. and Seddon, J. 1996, 'The social body and the biomechanical body: can they coexist in nurse education?', *The Journal of Advanced Medicine*, 23, pp. 651–656.

Brunskell-Evans, H. and Moore, M. (eds). 2018, *Transgender Children and Young People: Born in Your Own Body*, Cambridge Scholars Publishing, UK.

Burckhardt, C. S., Clark, S. R. and Bennett, R. M. 1993, 'Fibromyalgia and quality of life: a comparative analysis', *The Journal of Rheumatology*, 20(3), pp. 475–479.

Bury, M. 2001, 'Illness narratives: fact or fiction?', *Sociology of Health and Illness*, 23 (3), pp. 263–285.

Busse, J. W., Kulkarni, A. V., Badwall, P. and Guyatt, G. H. 2008, 'Attitudes towards fibromyalgia: a survey of Canadian chiropractic, naturopathic, physical therapy and occupational therapy students', *BMC Complementary and Alternative Medicine*, 8 (24), doi:10.1186/1472-6882-8-24.

Buytendijk, F. J. J. 1971, *Pain*, Greenwood Press, USA.

Canguilhem, G. 1991, *The Normal and the Pathological*, Zone Books, USA.

Canguilhem, G. 2008, *Knowledge of Life*, Fordham University Press, USA.

Caplan, A. 1992, 'Does the philosophy of medicine exist?', *Theoretical Medicine and Bioethics*, 13(1), pp. 67–77.

Carel, H. 2007, 'Can I be ill and happy?', *Philosophia*, 35(2), pp. 95–110.

Carel, H. 2008, *Illness: The Cry of the Flesh*, Acumen Publishing, UK.

Carel, H. 2013, 'Illness, phenomenology and philosophical method', *Theoretical Medicine and Bioethics*, 34(4), pp. 345–357.

Carel, H. 2014, 'The philosophical role of illness', *Metaphilosophy*, 45(1), pp. 20–40.

Carel, H. 2016a, 'The philosophical role of illness – and how it can teach us to live reflectively', *The Conversation*, retrieved from https://theconversation.com/the-philosophical-role-of-illness-and-how-it-can-teach-us-to-live-reflectively-57310

Carel, H. 2016b, *Phenomenology of Illness*, Oxford University Press, UK.

Carel, H. 2016c, 'Living in the present: illness, phenomenology, and well-being', Jackson, M. (Ed.) *The Routledge History of Disease*, Routledge, UK, pp. 581–599.

Carel, H. and Cooper, R. 2013, 'Introduction', in H. Carel and R. Cooper (eds), *Health, Illness and Disease*, Acumen Publishing, UK.

Carel, H., Kidd, I. J. and Pettigrew, R. 2016, 'Illness as transformative experience', *The Lancet*, 338(10050), p. 1153.

Charmaz, K. 1993, *Good Days, Bad Days: The Self in Chronic Illness and Time*, Rutgers University Press, USA.

Charon, R. 2008, *Narrative Medicine: Honouring the Stories of Illness*, Oxford University Press, UK.

Chinn, S., Caldwell, W. and Gritsenko, K. 2016, 'Fibromyalgia pathogenesis and treatment options update', *Current Pain and Headache Reports*, 20, p. 25.

Clark, C. D. 2012, 'Asthma episodes: stigma, children, and Hollywood films', *Medical Anthropology Quarterly*, 26, Issue 1, pp. 92–115.

Clark, P., Paiva, E. S., Ginovker, A. and Salomón, P. A. 2013, 'A patient and physician survey of fibromyalgia across Latin America and Europe', *BMC Musculoskeletal Disorders*, 14(188), doi:10.1186/1471-2474-14-188.

Clarke, B. 2012, 'Causation in medicine', in W. J. Gonzalez (ed.), *Conceptual Revolutions: from Cognitive Science to Medicine*, Netbiblo, Spain.

Clarke, J. N. and James, S. 2003, 'The radicalized self: the impact on the self of the contest nature of the diagnosis of chronic fatigue syndrome', *Social Science and Medicine*, 57, pp. 1387–1395.

Clauw, D. J. 2014, 'Fibromyalgia: a clinical review', *The Journal of the American Medical Association*, 311(154), pp. 1547–1555

Coady, D. 2010, 'Two concepts of epistemic injustice', *Episteme*, 7, pp. 101–113.

Cooper, R. '2002, Disease', *Studies in History and Philosophy of Science Part C: Studies in History and Philosophy of Biological and Biomedical Sciences*, 33(2), pp. 263–282.

Crowley-Matoka, M. *et al.* 2009, 'Problems of quality and equity in pain management: exploring the role of biomedical culture', *Pain Medicine*, 10(7), pp. 1312–1324.

Cunnien, A. J. 1997, 'Psychiatric and medical syndromes associated with deception', Rogers, R. (ed.) *Clinical Assessment of Malingering and Deception*, 2nd edition, The Guilford Press, USA, p. 23–46.

Daneshjou, K., Jafareih, H. and Raaeskarami, S. 2012, 'Congenital insensitivity to pain and anhydrosis (CIPA); a report of 4 cases', *The Iran Journal of Paediatrics*, 22 (3), pp. 412–416.

Darker, C., Casey, E.Seraukina, T., Whiston, L. and O'Shea, B. 2014, *The Patients' Perspective: A Survey of Chronic Disease Management in Ireland*, Report, Department of Public Health and Primary Care, Trinity College, Dublin.

Davis, B. and Vanderah, T. W. 2016, 'A new paradigm for pain', *The Journal of Family Practice*, 65(9), pp. 598–605.

Deep, P. 1999, 'Biological and biopsychosocial models of health and disease in dentistry', *The Journal of the Canadian Dental Association*, 65, pp. 496–497.

Denise, E. J. *et al.* 2012, 'Conditions comorbid with chronic fatigue in a population-based sample', *Psychosomatics*, 53(1), pp. 44–50.

De Vreese, L. 2016, 'Rethinking the concept of disease debate: a pragmatist alternative', unpublished manuscript.

Demitrack, M. A. 1998, 'Chronic fatigue syndrome and fibromyalgia: dilemmas in diagnosis and clinical management', *Psychiatric Clinics of North America*, 21(3), pp. 671–692.

Diaz-Piedra, C., Di Stasi, L. L., Baldwin, C. M., Buela-Casal, G. and Catena, A. 2015, 'Sleep disturbances of adult women suffering from fibromyalgia: a systematic review of observational studies', *Sleep Medicine Reviews*, 21, pp. 86–99.

Dobkin, P. L. *et al.* 2003, 'Patient–physician discordance in fibromyalgia', *The Journal of Rheumatology*, 30, pp. 1326–1334.

Douglas, H. E. 2009, *Science, Policy, and the Value-Free Ideal*, University of Pittsburgh Press, USA.

Dumit, J. 2006, 'Illnesses you have to fight to get: facts as forces in uncertain, emergent illnesses', *Social Science and Medicine*, 62, pp. 577–590.

Dupré, J. 1995, *The Disorder of Things: Metaphysical Foundations of the Disunity of Science*, Harvard University Press, USA.

Dusenbery, M. 2018, *Doing Harm*, HarperCollins, New York.

Edlich, R. F., Cross, C. L., Wack, C. A. and Long, W. B. 2009, 'Delusions of parasitosis', *The American Journal of Emergency Medicine*, 27(8), pp. 997–999.

Ehrlich, G. E. 2003, 'Pain is real; fibromyalgia isn't', *The Journal of Rheumatology*, 30 (8), pp. 1666–1667

Elliott, C. 2000, 'A New Way to Be Mad', *The Atlantic*, December.

Elliott, C. 2004, *Better Than Well: American Medicine Meets the American Dream*, W. W. Norton and Company, USA.

Elliott, C. 2011, *White Coat Black Hat: Adventures on the Dark Side of Medicine*, Beacon Press, USA.

Engel, G. L. 1977, 'The need for a new medical model: a challenge for biomedicine', *Science*, 196(4286), pp. 129–136.

Epstein, S. 1996, *Impure Science: AIDS, Activism, and the Politics of Knowledge*, University of California Press, USA.

Ereshefsky, M. 2009, 'Defining "health" and "disease"', *Studies in History and Philosophy of Biological and Biomedical Sciences*, 40(3), pp. 221–227.

Ferry-Danini, J. 2018, 'Should phenomenological approaches to illness be wary of naturalism?', *Studies of the History and Philosophy of Biological and Biomedical Sciences*, in press.

Fleck, L. 1981, *Genesis and Development of a Scientific Fact*, University of Chicago Press, USA.

Fleming, K. C. and Volcheck, M. M. 2015, 'Central sensitisation syndrome and the initial evaluation of a patient with fibromyalgia: a review', *Rambam Maimonides Medical Journal*, 6(2), e0020.

Floridi, L. 2011, *The Philosophy of Information*, Oxford University Press, UK.

Folks, D. G. 1995, 'Munchausen's syndrome and other factitious disorders', *Neurologic Clinics*, 13(2), pp. 267–281.

Ford, C. V. 1997, 'Somatization and fashionable diagnoses: illness as a way of life', *The Scandinavian Journal of Work and Environmental Health*, 23, Supp. 3, pp. 7–16.

Foucault, M. 1996, *The Birth of the Clinic: An Archaeology of Medical Perception*, Vintage, UK.

Franck, T. M. 2000, *The Empowered Self: Law and Society in an Age of Individualism*, Oxford University Press, UK.

Frank, A. 2013, *The Wounded Storyteller*, University of Chicago Press, USA.

Freudenmann, R. W. and Lepping, P. 2009, 'Delusional infestation', *Clinical Microbiology Reviews*, 22(4), pp. 690–732.

Fricker, M. 2007, *Epistemic Injustice: Power and the ethics of knowing*, Oxford University Press, UK.

Fukuda, K. 1994, 'The chronic fatigue syndrome: a comprehensive approach to its definition and study. International Chronic Fatigue Syndrome Study Group', *Annals of Internal Medicine*, 121(12), pp. 953–959.

Furnham, A. and Telford, K. 2012, 'Public attitudes, lay theories and mental health literacy: the understanding of mental health', in L. L'Abate (ed.), *Mental Illnesses: Understanding, Prediction and Control*, InTech, doi:10.5772/29413.

Ghazan-Shahi, S., Towheed, T. and Hopman, W. 2012, 'Should rheumatologists retain ownership of fibromyalgia? A survey of Ontario rheumatologists', *Clinical Rheumatology*, 31(8), pp. 1177–1181.

Giacomelli, C., Sernissi, F., Rossi, A., Bombardieri, S. and Bazzichi, L. 2014, 'Biomarkers in fibromyalgia: a review', *Current Biomarker Findings*, 4, pp. 35–41.

Glenton, C. 2003, 'Chronic back pain sufferers – striving for the sick role', *Social Science and Medicine*, 57, pp. 2243–2252.

Goffman, E. 1961, *Asylums: Essays on the Social Situation of Mental Patients and Other Inmates*, Doubleday Anchor, USA.

Goffman, E. 1968, *Stigma: Notes on the Management of Spoiled Identity*, Penguin, UK.

Goffman, E. 1969, 'The insanity of place', *Psychiatry: Journal of Interpersonal Relations*, 32(4), pp. 357–387.

Goldacre, B. 2012, *Bad Pharma: How Drug Companies Mislead Doctors and Harm Patients*, Fourth Estate, UK.

Goldberg, D. S. 2017, 'Pain, objectivity and history: understanding pain stigma', *Medical Humanities*, 43, pp. 238–243.

Goldenberg, D. L. 2009, *Clinical Management of Fibromyalgia*, Professional Communications, USA.

Goldenberg, D. L. *et al.* 2008, 'Understanding fibromyalgia and its related disorders', *Primary Care Companion to the Journal of Clinical Psychiatry*, 10(2), pp. 133–144.

Gordon, D. 1988, 'Tenacious assumptions in modern medicine', in D. Gordon and M. Lock (eds), *Biomedicine Examined*, Kluwer Academic Publishers, The Netherlands, pp. 19–56.

Greiffenstein, M. and Baker, J. 2005, 'Miller was (mostly) right: head injury severity inversely related to simulation', *Legal and Criminological Psychology*, 11, pp. 131–145.

Greve, K. W., Ord, J. S., Bianchini, K. J. and Curtis, K. L. 2009, 'Prevalence of malingering in patients with chronic pain referred for psychologic evaluation in a medico-legal context', *Archives of Physical Medicine and Rehabilitation*, 90(7), pp. 1117–1126.

Groch, S. 2001, 'Free Spaces: Creating Oppositional Consciousness in the Disability Rights Movement', in J. Mansbridge and A. Morris (eds), *Oppositional Consciousness: The Subjective Roots of Social Protest*, The University of Chicago Press, USA.

Hacking, I. 1991, 'A tradition of natural kinds', *Philosophical Studies*, 61(1), pp. 109–126.

Hacking, I. 1996, 'The Looping Effects of Human Kinds', in D. Sperber, D. Premack and A. J. Premack (eds), *Causal Cognition: A Multi-disciplinary Debate*, The Clarendon Press, Oxford, p. 351.

Hacking, I. 1998, *Rewriting the Soul: Multiple Personality and the Sciences of Memory*, Princeton University Press, USA.

Hacking, I. 1999, *The Social Construction of What?*, Harvard University Press, USA.

Hacking, I. 2002, *Mad Travelers*, Harvard University Press, USA.

Hacking, I. 2004, 'Between Michel Foucault and Erving Goffman: between discourse in the abstract and face-to-face interaction', *Economy and Society*, 33(3), pp. 277–302.

Hacking, I. 2006, 'Kinds of people: moving targets', The Tenth British Academy Lecture.

Hacking, I. 2009, 'Holberg Prize Lecture', The Holberg Prize Symposium.

Hadler, N. M. 2003, 'Editorial: "fibromyalgia" and the medicalisation of misery', *The Journal of Rheumatology*, 30(8), p. 1669.

Hall, R. C. W. and Hall, R. C. W. 2012, 'Compensation neurosis: a too quickly forgotten concept?', *The Journal of the American Academy of Psychiatry and the Law*, 40, pp. 390–398.

Hanh, S. R. *et al.* 1994, 'The difficult doctor–patient relationship: Somatization, personality and psychopathology', *Journal of Clinical Epidemiology*, 47(6), pp. 647–657.

Harth, M. and Nielson, W. R. 2014, 'Fibromyalgia and disability adjudication: No simple solutions to a complex problem', *Pain Research and Management*, 19(6), pp. 293–299.

Harth, M. 2013, 'Cursing the darkness: reactions to fibromyalgia', *Pain Research and Management*, 18(2), pp. 64–66.

Häuser, W., Wilhelm, R., Klein, W. and Zimmer, C. 2006, 'Causal illness attributions and healthcare utilization in fibromyalgia syndrome', *Der Schmerz*, 20(2), pp. 119–127.

Hayes, S. M. *et al.* 2010, 'Fibromyalgia and the therapeutic relationship: where uncertainty meets attitude', *Pain Research and Management*, 15(6), pp. 385–391.

Healy, D. 2004, *Let Them Eat Prozac*, New York University Press, USA.

Healy, D. 2012, *Pharmageddon*, University of California Press, USA.

Heidegger, M. 1978, *Being and Time*, Wiley-Blackwell, USA.

Heidsieck, A. 2007, 'Bellow, Styron, Roth: representation of anti-Semitism and its relationship to German cultural history in Jewish and non-Jewish American novels', inK. M. Bogdal, K. Holz and M. Lorenz (eds), *Literarischer Antisemitismus nach Auschwitz*, Metzler, Germany.

Hein, G. and Singer, T. 2008, 'I feel how you feel but not always: the empathic brain and its modulation', *Current Opinion in Neurobiology*, 18, pp. 153–158.

Helman, C. G. 1988, 'Psyche, soma, and society: the social construction of psychosomatic disorders', in D. Gordon and M. Lock (eds), *Biomedicine Examined*, Kluwer Academic Publishers, The Netherlands, pp. 95–122.

Hench, P. K. 1976, 'Nonarticular rheumatism, 22nd rheumatism review: review of the American and English literature for the years 1973 and 1974', *Arthritis and Rheumatism*, 19, pp. 1081–1089.

Henriksson, C. M., Liedberg, G. M. and Gerdle, B. 2005, 'Women with FM: work and rehabilitation', *Disability and Rehabilitation*, 27(12), pp. 685–695.

Hesslow, G. 1993, 'Do we need a concept of disease?', *Theoretical Medicine*, 14(1), pp. 1–14.

Hewitson, P. *et al.* 2014, 'People with limiting long-term conditions report poorer experiences and more problems with hospital care', *BMC Health Services Research*, 14(33).

Hoffman, D. L. and Dukes, E. M. 2008, 'The health status burden of people with fibromyalgia: a review of studies that assessed health status with the SF-36 or the SF-12 in *The International Journal of Clinical Practice*, 62(1), pp. 115–126.

Hofmann, B. 2002, 'On the triad disease, illness and sickness', *The Journal of Medical Philosophy*, 27(6), pp. 651–673.

Homma, M., Ishikawa, H. and Kiuchi, T. 2016, 'Association of Physicians' illness perception of fibromyalgia with frustration and resistance to accepting patients: a cross-sectional study', *Clinical Rheumatology*, 35(4), pp. 1019–1027.

Hookway, C. 2010, 'Some varieties of epistemic injustice: response to Fricker', *Episteme*, 7, pp. 151–163.

Hossenbaccus, Z. and White, P. D. 2013, 'Views on the nature of chronic fatigue syndrome: content analysis', *The JRSM Short Reports*, 4(4).

Husserl, E. 2012, *Ideas: General Introduction to Pure Phenomenology*, Routledge, UK.

Hylwa, S. A., Foster, A. A., Bury, J. E., Davis, M. D., Pittelkow, M. R. and Bostwick, J. M. 2012, 'Delusional infestation is typically comorbid with other psychiatric diagnoses: review of 54 patients receiving psychiatric evaluation at Mayo Clinic', *Psychosomatics*, 53(3), pp. 258–265.

Illari, P. and Russo, F. 2014, *Causality: Philosophical Theory meets Scientific Practice*, Oxford University Press, UK.

Impey, C., Buxner, S., Antonellis, J., Johnson, E. and King, C. 2011, 'A twenty-year survey of science literacy among college undergraduates', *The Journal of College Science Teaching*, 40(4), pp. 31–37.

Inanici, F. and Yunus, M. B. 2004, 'History of fibromyalgia: past to present', *Current Pain and Headache Reports*, 8, pp. 369–378.

Iverson, S. A., Howard, K. B. and Penney, B. K. 2008, 'Impact of internet use on health-related behaviours and the patient-physician relationship: a survey-based study and review', *The Journal of the American Osteopathic Association*, 108(12), pp. 699–711.

Jason, L. A., Taylor, R. R. *et al.* 2002, 'Evaluating attributions for an illness based upon the name: chronic fatigue syndrome, myalgic encephalopathy and Florence Nightingale disease', *The American Journal of Community Psychology*, 30(1), pp. 133–148.

Jensen, T. and Tyler, I. 2015, '"Benefits broods": the cultural and political crafting of anti-welfare commonsense', *Critical Social Policy*, 35(4), pp. 470–491.

Johnson, S. B. 2012, 'Medicine's paradigm shift: an opportunity for psychology', *The American Psychological Association*, 43(8), p. 5.

Johnson-Greene, D., Brooks, L. and Ference, T. 2013, 'Relationship between performance validity testing, disability status and somatic complaints in patients with fibromyalgia', *Clinical Neuropsychology*, 27(1), pp. 148–158.

Jones, M. A. 2003, 'Laws, lies, and videotape: malingering as a legal phenomenon', in P. W. Halligan and C. Bass (eds), *Malingering and Illness Deception*, Oxford University Press, UK, pp. 209–219.

Jung, B. and Reidenberg, M. M. 2007, 'Physicians being deceived', *Pain Medicine*, 8 (5), pp. 433–437.

Jutel, A. 2009, 'Sociology of diagnosis: a preliminary review', *Sociology of Health of Illness*, 31(2), pp. 278–299.

Jutel, A. 2011, *Putting a Name to It: Diagnosis in Contemporary Society*, Johns Hopkins University Press, USA.

Jutel, A. 2015, 'Beyond the sociology of diagnosis', *Sociology Compass*, 9(9), pp. 841–852.

Kaminer, W. 2000, *Sleeping With Extra-Terrestrials: The Rise of Irrationalism and Perils of Piety*, Vintage, UK.

Kaplan, R. M., Schmidt, S. M. and Cronan, T. A. 2000, 'Quality of well being in patients with fibromyalgia', *The Journal of Rheumatology*, 27(3), pp. 785–789.

Keating, P. and Cambrosio, A. 2003, *Biomedical Platforms: Realigning the Normal and the Pathological in Late-Twentieth-Centure Medicine*, The MIT Press, USA.

Khushf, G. 2007, 'An agenda for future debate on concepts of health and disease', *Medicine, Health Care and Philosophy*, 10, pp. 19–27.

Kidd, I. J. 2012, 'Can illness be edifying?', *Inquiry*, 55(5), pp. 496–520.

Kidd, I. J. and Carel, H. 2017, 'Epistemic injustice and illness', *The Journal of Applied Philosophy*, 34(2), doi:10.1111/japp.12172.

Kingma, E. 2013, 'Health and disease: social constructivism as a combination of naturalism and normativism', in H. Carel and R. Cooper (eds), *Health, Illness and Disease*, Acumen Publishing, UK.

Kingma, E. 2014, 'Naturalism about health and disease: adding nuance for progress', *The Journal of Medicine and Philosophy*, 39, pp. 590–608.

Kingma, E. 2017, 'Disease as scientific and as value-laden concept', in T. Schramme and S. Edwards (eds), *Handbook of the Philosophy of Medicine*, Springer, Germany, pp. 45–63.

Kirmayer, L. J. 1988, 'Mind and body as metaphors: hidden values in biomedicine', in D. Gordon and M. Lock (eds), *Biomedicine Examined*, Kluwer Academic Publishers, The Netherlands, pp. 57–93.

Kitwood, T. 2002, 'Towards the reconstruction of an organic mental disorder', in A. Radley (ed.), *Worlds of Illness: Biographical and Cultural Perspectives on Health and Disease*, Routledge, UK.

Kleinman, A. 1988, *The Illness Narratives*, Basic Books, USA.

Kraag, G. 'Fibromyalgia', in Mosher, D., Stein, H. and Kraag, G. (eds). 2002, *Living Well with Arthritis*, Viking Press, Canada, pp. 55–64.

Kralik, D., Brown, M. and Koch, T. 2001, 'Women's experiences of "being diagnosed" with a long-term illness', *The Journal of Advanced Nursing*, 33(5), pp. 594–602.

Kravitz, H. M. and Katz, R. S. 2015, 'Fibrofog and fibromyalgia: a narrative review and implications', *Rheumatology International*, 35, pp. 1115–1125.

Kroll-Smith, S. and Floyd, H. 1997, *Bodies in Protest: Environmental Illness and the Struggle over Medical Knowledge*, New York University Press, USA.

Kuorikoski, J. and Pöyhönen, S. 2012, 'Looping kinds and social mechanisms', *Sociological Theory*, 30(3), pp. 187–205.

Kuperman, V. 2006, 'Narratives of psychiatric malingering in works of fiction', *The Journal of Medical Ethics; Medical Humanities*, 32, pp. 67–72.

Lacourt, T., Houtveen, J. and van Doornen, L. 2013, '"Functional somatic syndromes, one or many?": an answer by cluster analysis', *The Journal of Psychosomatic Research*, 74(1), pp. 6–11.

Lane, H. 1999, *The Mask of Benevolence: Disabling the Deaf Community*, Dawn Sign Press, USA.

Lane, C. 2008, *Shyness: How Normal Behaviour Became a Sickness*, Yale University Press, USA.

Larkin, M. 1998, 'Elaine Showalter: hysteria's historian', *The Lancet*, 351(9116), p. 1638.

Latour, B. 1987, *Science in Action*, Harvard University Press, USA.

Latour, B. 1999, *Pandora's Hope: Essays on the Reality of Science Studies*, Harvard University Press, USA.

Latour, B. 2004, 'Why has critique run out of steam? From matters of fact to matters of concern', *Critical Inquiry*, 30(2), pp. 225–248.

Latour, B. and Woolgar, S. 1986, *Laboratory Life: The Construction of Scientific Facts*, Princeton University Press, USA.

Lawler, J. 1991, *Behind the Screens: Nursing, Somology and the Problem of the Body*, Churchill Livingstone, Australia.

Leder, D. 1990, *The Absent Body*, University of Chicago Press, USA.

Ledford, D. K. and Lockey, R. F. 2013, 'Asthma and comorbidities', *Current Opinion in Allergy and Clinical Immunology*, 13(1), pp. 78–86.

Lee, J. W. *et al.* 2017, 'Determinants of quality of life in patients with fibromyalgia: a structural equation modelling approach', *PLoS ONE*, 12(2), e0171186. doi:10.1371/journal.pone.0171186.

Lemoine, M. 2013, 'Defining disease beyond conceptual analysis: an analysis of conceptual analysis in philosophy of medicine', *Theoretical Medicine and Bioethics*, 34 (4), pp. 309–325.

Lessing, D. 2007, *The Golden Notebook*, Harper Perennial, UK.

Levin, E. C. and Gieler, U. 2013, 'Delusions of parasitosis', *Seminars in Cutaneous Medicine and Surgery*, 32(2), pp. 73–77.

Lilienfeld, S. O. and Marino, L. 1995, 'Mental disorder as a Roschian concept: a critique of Wakefield's "harmful dysfunction analysis"', *The Journal of Abnormal Psychology*, 104(3), pp. 411–420.

Lindell, L., Bergman, S., Petersson, I. F., Jacobsson, L. T. H., and Herrstrom, P. 2000, 'Prevalence of fibromyalgia and chronic widespread pain', *Scandinavian Journal of Primary Health Care*, 18(3), pp. 149–153.

Lippel, K. 2008, 'Workers' compensation and controversial illnesses', in P. Moss and K. Teghtsoonian (eds), *Contesting Illness: Process and Practices*, University of Toronto Press, Canada.

Lis, E. 2015, 'His Majesty's psychosis: the case of Emperor Joshua Norton', *Academic Psychiatry*, 39(2), pp. 181–185.

Löfgren, M., Ekholm, J. and Öhman, A. 2006, '"A constant struggle": successful strategies of women in work despite FM', *Disability and Rehabilitation*, 28(7), pp. 447–455.

MacKenzie, D. 1990, *Inventing Accuracy: A Historical Sociology of Nuclear Missile Guidance*, MIT Press, USA.

MacKenzie, D. 1998, 'The certainty trough', in R. Williams, W. Faulkner and J. Fleck (eds), *Exploring Expertise*, Palgrave Macmillan, UK.

Macnicol, J. 2011, 'The history of work-disability in the UK, from the 1880s to the 1950s', Social Policy Association Conference, 4–6 July, University of Lincoln.

Madden, S. and Sim, J. 2016, 'Acquiring a diagnosis of fibromylagia syndrome: The sociology of diagnosis', in *Social Theory & Health*, 14(1), pp. 88–108.

Main, S. 2014, 'Picturing pain: using creative methods to communicate the experience of chronic pain', *Pain News*, 12(1), pp. 32–35.

Malleson, A. 2002, *Whiplash and Other Useful Illnesses*, McGill-Queen's University Press, Canada.

Mansbridge, J. J. 2001, 'The making of oppositional consciousness' in J. J. Mansbridge and A. Morris (eds), *Oppositional Consciousness: The Subjective Roots of Social Protest*, University of Chicago Press, USA, pp. 1–19.

Marinka, M. 1975, 'Why make people patients', *The Journal of Medical Ethics*, 1, pp. 81–84.

Marmot, M., Allen, J., Goldblatt, P. *et al.* 2010, *Healthy Lives, Brighter Futures: The Strategy for Children and Young People's Health*, Marmot Review Team, UK.

Matthias, M. S. and Bair, M. J. 2010, 'The patient–provider relationship in chronic pain management: where do we go from here?', *Pain Medicine*, 11(12), pp. 1747–1749.

Mayne, P., English, J. S., Kilbane, E. J, Burke, J. M., Middelveen, M. J. and Stricker, R. 2013, 'Morgellons: a novel dermatological perspective as the multisystem infective disease borreliosis', *F1000Research*, 2(118), doi:10.12688/f1000research.2–118.v1.

McCartney, M. 2012, 'Medicine and the media: Atos and changes to disabled people's benefits', *The British Medical Journal*, 344(7844), p. 30.

Merleau-Ponty, M. 2013, *Phenomenology of Perception*, Routledge, UK.

Mishler, E. G. 1984, *The Discourse of Medicine: Dialectics of Medical Interviews*, Ablex, USA.

Moes-Wójtowicz, A. *et al.* 2012, 'Asthma as a psychosomatic disorder: the causes, scale of the problem, and the association with alexithymia and disease control', *Pneumonologia i Alergologia Polska*, 80(1), pp. 13–19.

Mol, A. 2003, *The Body Multiple*, Duke University Press, USA.

Mol, A. and Law, J. 2007, 'Embodied action, enacted bodies', in R. V. Burri and J. Dumit (eds), *Biomedicine as Culture: Instrumental Practices, Technoscientific Knowledge and New Modes of Life*, Routledge, UK, pp. 88–89.

Mold, A. 2010, 'Patient groups and the construction of the patient-consumer in Britain: an historical overview', *The Journal of Social Policy*, 39(4), pp. 505–521.

Mold, A. 2015, 'Making British patients into consumers', *The Lancet*, 385(9975), pp. 1286–1287.

Moldofsky, H., Scarisbrick, P., England, R. and Smythe, H.1978, 'Musculoskeletal symptoms and non-REM sleep disturbance in patients with "fibrositis" syndrome', *Bulletin on the Rheumatological Diseases*, 28, pp. 928–931.

Moore, L. 2008, *The Collected Stories*, Faber & Faber, UK.

Moran, D. 1999, *Introduction to Phenomenology*, Routledge, UK.

Mullan, F. 1986, 'Revolt of the postmodern patient', *The New York Times*, 2 February.

Muramatsu, Y. *et al.* 2001, 'Bronchial asthma: psychosomatic aspect', *The Journal of the Japan Medical Association*, 126(3), pp. 375–377.

Neerinckx, E., van Houdenhove, B., Lysens, R., Vertommen, H. and Onghena, P. 2000, 'Attributions in chronic fatigue syndrome and fibromyalgia syndrome in tertiary care', *The Journal of Rheumatology*, 27(4), pp. 1051–1055.

Neilson, S. 2016, 'Pain as metaphor: metaphor and medicine', *Medical Humanities*, 42, pp. 3–10.

Nettleton, S. 2006, *The Sociology of Health and Illness*, Polity Press, UK.

NICE. 2007, *Chronic Fatigue Syndrome/Myalgic Encephalomyelitis (or Encephalopathy): Diagnosis and Management of CFS in Adults and Children*, National Institute of Clinical Excellence, UK.

Nordenfelt, L. 2013, 'The opposition between naturalistic and holistic theories of health and disease', in H. Carel and R. Cooper (eds), *Health, Illness and Disease*, Acumen Publishing, UK.

Oreskes, N. and Conway, E. M. 2011, *Merchants of Doubt: How a Handful of Scientists Obscured the Truth on Issues from Tobacco Smoke to Global Warming*, Bloomsbury Press, UK.

O'Sullivan, S. 2015, *It's All in Your Head: True Stories of Imaginary Illness*, Chatto and Windus, UK.

Padfield, D. and Zakrewska, J. M. 2017, 'Encountering pain', *The Lancet*, 389, pp. 1177–1178.

Padfield, D., Zakrzewska, J. M. and Williams, A. C. C. 2015, 'Do photographic images of pain improve communication during pain consultations?', *Pain Research and Management*, 20(3), pp. 123–128.

Palmer, I. P. 2003, 'Malingering, shirking and self-inflicted injuries in the military', in P. W. Halligan and C. Bass (eds), *Malingering and Illness Deception*, Oxford University Press, UK, pp. 42–53.

Pankratz, L. and Erickson, R. C. 1990, 'Two views of malingering', *Clinical Neuropsychologist*, 4(4), pp. 379–389.

Parsons, T. 1951, *The Social System*, Routledge, UK.

Parsons, T. and Fox, R. 1952, 'Illness, therapy and the modern urban American family', in E. Jaco (ed.), *Patients Physicians and Illness*, The Free Press, USA.

Paul, L. A. 2014, *Transformative Experience*, Oxford University Press, UK.

Pearson, M. L., Selby, J. V., Cantrell, V., Braden, C. R. *et al.* 2012, 'Clinical, epidemiologic, histopathologic and molecular features of an unexplained dermopathy', *PLoS ONE* 7(1): e29908. doi:10.1371/journal.pone.0029908.

Pendsey, S. P. 2010, 'Understanding diabetic foot', *The International Journal of Diabetes in Developing Countries*, 30(2), pp. 75–79.

Perring, C. 1997, 'Review: *Hystories*', *Metapsychology*, 1(27).

Perrot, S., Choy, E., Petersel, D., Ginovker, A. and Kramer, E. 2012, 'Survey of physician experiences and perceptions about the diagnosis and treatment of fibromyalgia', *British Medical Council Health Services Research*, 12(356), doi: 10.1186/1472-6963-12-356.

Piccirillo, J. F. *et al.* 2008, 'The changing prevalence of comorbidity across the age spectrum', *Critical Reviews in Oncology/Haematology*, 67(2), pp. 124–132.

Polonsky, K. S. 2012, 'The past 200 years in diabetes', *The New England Journal of Medicine*, 367, pp. 1332–1340.

Porter, R. 2002, *Blood and Guts: A Short History of Medicine*, Penguin Books, UK.

Price, J. R., Mitchell, E., Tidy, E. and Hunot, V. 2008, 'Cognitive behavioural therapy for chronic fatigue syndrome in adults', *Cochrane Database of Systematic Reviews*, 3, article CD001027.

Prince, M. J. 2008, 'Claiming a disability benefit as contesting social citizenship', in P. Moss and K. Teghtsoonian (eds), *Contesting Illness: Process and Practices*, University of Toronto Press, Canada.

Queiroz, L. P. 2013, 'Worldwide epidemiology of fibromyalgia', *Current Pain and Headache Reports*, 17(356).

Quirke, V. and Gaudillière, J. 2008, 'The era of biomedicine: science, medicine, and public health in Britain and France after the Second World War', *Medical History*, 52, pp. 442–443.

Radley, A. 1994, *Making Sense of Illness: the Social Psychology of Health and Disease*, Sage, UK.

Raine, A. 2003, 'Malingering and criminal behaviour as psychopathology', in P. W. Halligan and C. Bass (eds), *Malingering and Illness Deception*, Oxford University Press, UK, pp. 93–106.

Reznek, L. 1987, *The Nature of Disease*, Routledge and Kegan Paul, USA.

Robinson, I. 1990, 'Personal narratives, social careers and medical courses: analysing life trajectories in autobiographies of people with multiple sclerosis', *Social Science and Medicine*, 30(11), pp. 1173–1186.

Robinson, W. P. 2003, 'The contemporary cultural context for deception and malingering in Britain', in P. W. Halligan and C. Bass (eds), *Malingering and Illness Deception*, Oxford University Press, UK, pp. 132–146.

Rogers, R. and Neumann, C. S. 2003, 'Conceptual issues and explanatory models of malingering', in P. W. Halligan and C. Bass (eds), *Malingering and Illness Deception*, Oxford University Press, UK, pp. 71–82.

Rosen, G. M. and Taylor, S. 2007, 'Pseudo-PTSD', *Journal of Anxiety Disorders*, 21, pp. 201–210.

Sansone, R. A. and Sansone, L. A. 2012, 'Doctor shopping: a phenomenon of many themes', *Innovations in Clinical Neuroscience*, 9(11–12), pp. 42–46.

Sartre, J. 1969, *Being and Nothingness: The Complete Text*, Washington Square Press, USA.

Savely, V. R., Leitao, M. M. and Stricker, R. B. 2006, 'The mystery of morgellons disease: infection or delusion?', *American Journal of Clinical Dermatology*, 7(1), pp. 1–5.

Scadding, J. G. 1990, 'The semantic problems of psychiatry', *Psychological Medicine*, 20(2), pp. 243–248.

Scarry, E. 1985, *The Body in Pain: The Making and Unmaking of the World*, Oxford University Press, USA.

Schivelbusch, W. 2014, *The Railway Journey: The Industrialization of Time and Space in the Nineteenth Century, With a New Preface*, University of California Press, USA.

Schmaus, W. 1992, 'Sociology and Hacking'strousers', *PSA: Proceedings of the Biennial Meeting of the Philosophy of Science Association*, 1, pp. 167–173.

Schmelkin, L. 1988, 'Multidimensional perspectives in the perception of disabilities', in H. Yuker (ed.), *Attitudes toward Persons with Disabilities*, Springer, USA, pp. 127–137.

Schrag, C. O. 1982, 'Being in pain', in V. Kestenbaum (ed.), *The Humanity of the Ill*, University of Tennessee Press, USA, pp. 101–124.

Schramme, T. 2007, 'A qualified defence of a naturalist theory of health', *Medicine, Health Care and Philosophy*, 10, pp. 11–17.

Schwartz, P. H. 2007, 'Decision and discovery in defining "disease"', in H. Kincaid and J. McKitrick (eds), *Establishing Medical Reality: Essays in the Metaphysics and Epistemology of Biomedical Science*, Springer, UK.

Schwartz, P. H. 2014, 'Reframing the disease debate and defending the biostatistical theory', *The Journal of Medicine and Philosophy*, 39, pp. 572–589.

Scott, D. W. and Scott, L. C. 2003, *The Extremely Unfortunate Skull Valley Incident*, Trafford Publishing, USA.

Segall, A. 1976, 'The sick role concept: understanding illness behavior', *The Journal of Health and Social Behavior*, 17(2), pp. 162–169.

Shalin, D. N. 2014, 'Goffman on mental illness: asylums and "the insanity of place" revisited', *Symbolic Interaction*, 37(1), pp. 122–144.

Sharpe, M. 2003, 'Distinguishing malingering from psychiatric disorders', P. W. Halligan and C. Bass (eds), *Malingering and Illness Deception*, Oxford University Press, UK, pp. 156–170.

Sholl, J. 2015, 'Putting phenomenology in its place: some limits of a phenomenology of medicine', *Theoretical Medical Bioethics*, 36(6), pp. 391–410.

Shorter, E. 1986, *Bedside Manners: The Troubled History of Doctors and Patients*, Penguin Books, UK.

Shorter, E. 1993, *From Paralysis to Fatigue: A History of Psychosomatic Illness in the Modern Era*, The Free Press, USA.

Shorter, E. 1994, *From the Mind into the Body: The Cultural Origins of Psychosomatic Symptoms*, The Free Press, USA.

Showalter, E. 1997, *Hystories: Hysteria, Gender and Culture*, Pan Books Limited, UK.

Sigerist, H. 1936, 'History of medicine and the history of science: an open letter to George Sarton, editor of Isis', *The Bulletin of the History of Medicine*, 4, pp. 1–13.

Smart, B. 2016, *Concepts and Causes in the Philosophy of Disease*, Palgrave Macmillan, UK, pp. 22–42.

Smith, H. S., Harris, R. E., Clauw, D. J. 2011, 'Fibromyalgia', in H. T., Benzon, S. N. Raja, R. E. Molly, S. S. Liu and S. M. Fishman (eds), *Essentials of pain medicine*, 3rd ed., Elsevier, USA, pp. 345–350.

Smythe, H. 1972, 'Nonarticular rheumatism and psychogenic musculoskeletal syndromes', in D. J. McCarty (ed.), *Arthritis and Allied Conditions*, Lea and Febiger, USA, pp. 881–891.

Snyder, M. 2016, *Genomics & Personalized Medicine: What Everyone Needs To Know*, Oxford University Press, UK.

Solomon, M. 2015, *Making Medical Knowledge*, Oxford University Press, UK.

Sontag, S. 1978, *Illness as Metaphor*, Farrar, Straus, and Giroux, USA.

Spicker, S. F. 1987, 'An introduction to the medical epistemology of Georges Canguilhem: moving beyond Michel Foucault', *The Journal of Medical Philosophy*, 12 (4), pp. 397–411.

Sprince, A. 2003, 'Malingering and the law: a third way', in P. W. Halligan and C. Bass (eds), *Malingering and Illness Deception*, Oxford University Press, UK, pp. 232–242.

Starr, P. 1982, *The Social Transformation of American Medicine*, Basic Books, USA.

Stempsey, W. E. 2008, 'Philosophy of medicine is what philosophers of medicine do', *Perspectives in Biology and Medicine*, 51(3), pp. 379–391.

Stenhoff, A. L., Sadreddini, S., Peters, S. and Wearden, A. 2015, 'Understanding medical students' views of chronic fatigue syndrome: a qualitative study', *Journal of Health Psychology*, 20(2), pp. 198–209.

Stewart, D. C., and Sullivan, T. J. 1982, 'Illness behaviour and the sick role in chronic disease: the case of multiple sclerosis', *Social Science and Medicine*, 16(15), pp. 1397–1404.

Stone, J., Smyth, R., Carson, A., Warlow, C. and Sharpe, M. 2006, 'La belle indifférence in conversion symptoms and hysteria', *British Journal of Psychiatry*, 188, pp. 204–209.

Subbarao, P., Mandhane, P. J. and Sears, M. R. 2009, 'Asthma: epidemiology, etiology and risk factors', *Canadian Medical Association Journal*, 181(9), pp. 181–190.

Sullivan, M. 1986, 'In what sense is contemporary medicine dualistic?', *Culture, Medicine and Psychology*, 10(4), pp. 331–350

Svenaeus, F. 2017, *Phenomenological Bioethics: Medical Technologies, Human Suffering, and the Meaning of Being Alive*, Routledge, UK.

Swoboda, D. A. 2005, 'Embodiment and the search for illness legitimacy among women with contested illnesses', *Michigan Feminist Studies*, 19, pp. 73–90.

Swoboda, D. A. 2006, 'The social construction of contested illness legitimacy: a grounded theory analysis', *Qualitative Research in Psychology*, 3, pp. 233–251.

Tan, S. S. and Gonnawardene, N. 2017, 'Internet health information seeking and the patient-physician relationship: a systematic review', *The Journal of Medical Internet Research*, 19(1), e9.

Tekin, S. 2014, 'The missing self in Hacking's looping effects', in H. Kincaid and J. A. Sullivan (eds), *Classifying Psychopathology: Mental Kinds and Natural Kinds*, The MIT Press, USA.

Temkin, O. 1977, 'Health and disease', in his *The Double Face of Janus and Other Essays in the History of Medicine*, John Hopkins University Press, USA.

Theoharides, T. C., Tsilioni, I., Arbetman, L. *et al.* 2015, 'Fibromyalgia syndrome in need of effective treatments', *The Journal of Pharmacology and Experimental Therapeutics*, 355, pp. 255–263.

Thompson, J. 1977, 'Applause, applause', *Ploughshares*, 3(3–4), pp. 223–242.

Thrall, J. H. 2005, 'Prevalence and costs of chronic disease in a healthcare system structured for treatment of acute illness', *Radiology*, 235(1), pp. 9–12.

Time Magazine. 1960, 'Cuba: Castro's brain', *Time Magazine*, August.

Timmermans, S. and Haas, S. 2008, 'Towards a sociology of disease', *Sociology of Health and Illness*, 30(5), pp. 659–676.

Toombs, S. K. 1987, 'The meaning of illness: a phenomenological approach to the patient-physician relationship', *The Journal of Medicine and Philosophy*, 12, pp. 228–235.

Toombs, S. K. 1990, 'The temporality of illness: four levels of experience', *Theoretical Medicine*, 11, pp. 227–241.

Toombs, S. K. 1993, *The Meaning of Illness: A Phenomenological Account of the Different Perspectives of Physician and Patient*, Springer, USA.

Toombs, S. K. 1995, 'The lived experience of disability', *Human Studies*, 18, pp. 9–23.

Tveito, K. 2014, 'So many things we do not know', *Tidsskr Nor Legeforen (Journal of the Norwegian Medical Association)*, 11(134), pp. 1117–1178.

Twaddle, A. and Nordenfelt, L. (eds). 1993, *Disease, Illness and Sickness: Three Central Concepts in the Theory of Health*, Linköping University Press, Sweden.

Updike, J. 1970, *The Centaur*, Penguin Books, UK.

van Wilgen, C. P., van Ittersum, M. W., Kaptein, A. A. and van Wijhe, M. 2008, 'Illness perceptions in patients with fibromyalgia and their relationship to quality of life and catastrophizing', *Arthritis and Rheumatism*, 58(11), pp. 3618–3626.

Varul, M. Z. 2010, 'Talcott Parsons, the sick role and chronic illness', *Body & Society*, 16(2), pp. 72–94.

Vincent, A., Whipple, M. O. and McAllister, S. J. *et al.* 2015, 'A cross-sectional assessment of the prevalence of multiple chronic conditions and medication use in a sample of community-dwelling adults with fibromyalgia in Olmsted County, Minnesota', *BMJ Open*, 5, e006681. doi:10.1136/bmjopen-2014-006681.

von Engelhardt, D. 2008, 'How to support the patient with chronic disease: a philosophical point of view', *Journal of Nephrology*, 21(13), pp. 27–28.

Wade, D. T. and Halligan, P. W. 2004, 'Do biomedical models of illness make for good healthcare systems?', *The British Medical Journal*, 329(7479), p. 1398.

Wagner, E. H. 1998, 'Chronic disease management: what will it take to improve care for chronic illness?', *Effective Clinical Practice*, 1(1), pp. 2–4.

Wakefield, J. C. 1992, 'The concept of mental disorder', *American Psychologist*, 47(3), pp. 373–388.

Walker, C. 2001, 'Recognising the changing boundaries of illness in defining terms of chronic illness: a prelude to understanding the changing needs of people with chronic illness', *Australian Health Review*, 24(2), pp. 207–214.

Walker, E. A. *et al.* 1997, 'Predictors of physician frustration in the care of patients with rheumatological complaints', *General Hospital Psychiatry*, 19(5), pp. 315–323.

Wallman, K. E., Morton, A. R., Goodman, C., Grove, R. and Guilfoyle, A. M. 2004, 'Randomised controlled trial of graded exercise in chronic fatigue syndrome', *Medical Journal of Australia*, 180, pp. 444–448.

Wasan, A. D. *et al.* 2005, 'Dealing with difficult patients in your pain practice', *Regional Anesthesia and Pain Medicine*, 30(2), pp. 184–192.

Werner, A. and Malterud, K. 2003, 'It is hard work behaving as a credible patient: encounters between women with chronic pain and their doctors', *Social Science and Medicine*, 57, pp. 1409–1419.

Wessely, S. and Showalter, E. 1999, 'Chronic fatigue syndrome : a true illness or a social and political issue?', in G. Williams (ed.), *Horizons in Medicine, Vol. 10*, Royal College of Physicians, UK, pp. 501–516.

Wessely, S., Sharpe, M. and Nimnuan, C. 1999, 'Functional somatic syndromes: one or many?', *Lancet*, 354, pp. 936–939.

Wessely, S. and White, P. D. 2004, 'In debate: there is only one functional somatic syndrome', *The British Journal of Psychiatry*, 185(2), pp. 95–96.

Whitehead, L. 2006, 'Quest, chaos and restitution: living with chronic fatigue syndrome/myalgic encephalomyelitis', *Social Science and Medicine*, 62, pp. 2236–2245.

Whiting, P., Bagnall, A. M., Sowden, A. J., Cornell, J. E., Mulrow, C. D. and Ramirez, G. 2001, 'Interventions for the treatment and management of chronic fatigue syndrome: a systematic review', *The Journal of the American Medical Association*, 286, pp.1360–1368.

Wikman, A., Marklind, S. and Alexanderson, K. 2005, 'Illness, disease and sickness absence an empirical test of differences between concepts of ill health', *The Journal of Epidemiological Community Health*, 59, pp. 450–454.

Wittgenstein, L. 2009, *Philosophical Investigations*, 4th ed., Wiley-Blackwell, UK.

Wolfe, F. '2009, Fibromyalgia wars', *The Journal of Rheumatology*, 36, pp. 671–678.

Wolfe, F. and Walitt, B. 2013, 'Culture, science and the changing nature of fibromyalgia', *Nature Reviews Rheumatology*, 9, pp. 751–755.

Wolfe, F. *et al.* 2010, 'The American College of Rheumatology preliminary diagnostic criteria for fibromyalgia and measurement of symptom severity', *Arthritis Care and Research*, 62(5), pp. 600–610.

Wolfe, F., Smythe, H. A. and Yunus, M. B. 1990, 'The American College of Rheumatology 1990 criteria for the classification of fibromyalgia: report of the Multicenter Criteria Committee', *Arthritis and Rheumatism*, 33, pp. 160–172.

Wood, P. R. *et al.* 2002, 'Relationships between welfare status, health insurance status and health and medical care among children with asthma', *The American Journal of Public Health*, 92(9), pp. 1446–1452.

Woolf, V. 2002, *On Being Ill*, Paris Press, USA.

Wright, B. 1988, 'Attitudes and the fundamental negative bias: conditions and corrections', in H. Yuker (ed.), *Attitudes toward persons with disabilities*, Springer, USA, pp. 2–21.

Wright, L. 1973, 'Functions', *Philosophical Review*, 82, pp. 139–168.

Wynne, B. 1992, 'Uncertainty and environmental learning: reconceiving science and policy in the preventive paradigm', *Global Environmental Change*, 2(2), pp. 111–127.

Yunus, M. B. 1983, 'Fibromyalgia: a need for uniform classification', *The Journal of Rheumatology*, 10, pp. 841–844.

Yunus, M. B. 2011, 'The prevalence of fibromyalgia in other chronic pain conditions', *Pain Research and Treatment*, article 584573.

Yunus, M. B. 2015, 'Editorial review: an update on central sensitivity syndromes and the issues of nosology and psychobiology', *Current Rheumatology Reviews*, 11(2), pp. 70–85.

Index